THE
FOREVER
FACTOR

Add Years to Your Life, and Life to Your Years

Rhonda,
To a wonderful
lady. I hope you
enjoy this — you're
the best.
Dr B——

THE
FOREVER
FACTOR

Add Years to Your Life, and Life to Your Years

James J. Barber, M.D.

with Dorothy S. Casper
and Vicki C. Spackman

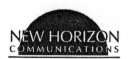

NEW HORIZON
COMMUNICATIONS

ISBN: 1-55517-696-8
e.1

Published by New Horizon Communications
An imprint of Cedar Fort, Inc.
www.cedarfort.com

Distributed by:

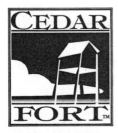

Typeset by Kristin Nelson
Cover design by Nicole Cunningham
Cover design © 2003 by Lyle Mortimer

Printed in the United States of America
10 9 8 7 6 5 4 3 2 1

Printed on acid-free paper

Library of Congress Cataloging-in-Publication Data

Barber, James J.
 The forever factor : add years to your life, and life to your years /
James J. Barber.
     p. cm.
Includes bibliographical references.
 ISBN 1-55517-696-8 (pbk. : alk. paper)
1. Longevity. I. Title.

 RA776.75.B363 2003
 612.6'8--dc21

                    2003002388

Disclaimer

The information and procedures contained in this book are based upon the research and the personal and professional experiences of the author. They are not intended as a substitute for consulting with your physician or other health care providers. The publisher and author are not responsible for any adverse effects or consequences resulting from the use of any of the suggestions, preparations, or procedures discussed in this book. All matters pertaining to your physical health should be supervised by a health care professional.

Foreword

As a midway member of the "Baby Boomer" generation, my attention is easily drawn to the concept of "anti-aging"—a belief that one can slow down and even reverse what has, until this past decade, been the unstoppable progression of time. Until the mid 1990s, we scientists were busy breaking the genetic code, determining new risk factors for cardiovascular disease, and developing new antiretroviral drugs to deal with the rising tide of HIV infections.

As the common medical problems of pneumonia have been largely controlled with new powerful antibiotics and diseases like polio and smallpox have essentially been eradicated from the planet via worldwide immunization programs, we can now turn our attention to discovering the secrets to slowing aging.

We are living longer than ever, almost doubling the life expectancy in most industrialized countries over the past one hundred years. Now our concerns are related to the diseases of aging (cancer, Alzheimer's disease, etc.) and, indeed, the process of aging. We have known for a while that there are multiple factors associated with aging—some genetic, but most related to our lifestyle, such as diet, weight, exercise, smoking, stress management, etc. These lifestyle factors are stronger determinants of the aging process than mere genetics.

So much is in our control. In this book, Dr. Barber presents strategies for you to take control of your destiny. He presents an extensive course on the theories of aging and specific ways in which you can slow down the aging process—through supplementation with herbs and specific nutrients, by certain stress management techniques, and by making lifestyle changes. The changes Dr. Barber suggests have the potential to add years to your life, and to help you look and feel younger than your chronological age. I know that you will find Dr. Barber's approach, as I have, enjoyable reading as well as life-changing! Start taking control of your aging process today. Optimize the quality of your life through the lessons you will learn as you read this book.

Embrace the possibilities!

Jamie McManus, MD, FAAFP
Los Angeles, California

Answers to Aging

A myriad of thoughts often crowd into our minds when certain words come into a conversation, such as "age" or "aging." Every year as high school and college reunions roll around, the first thoughts most of us have are, "How do I look? Do I look my age?"

The pattern of our growing-up years, family practices, and the rush hours of our lives become an impetus which encourages thoughts such as:

"We all get old, and there's nothing we can do about it."
"I'm too old to do that any more."
"Poor health is just a part of getting old."

We often see the end of our lives as an inevitable, downhill spiral.

However, Dr. James J. Barber, renowned in his field as a plastic surgeon, medical doctor, and anti-aging expert, knows that aging can be otherwise. He says:

We all have to age; however, the key is we do not have to age at the rate, time and the way we are doing it right now. There is a way to stop and even reverse some of the aging process.

Dr. Barber is a man who loves his work and loves people. He has a burning desire to help others and to make a difference. He is engaging and entertaining when he addresses an audience, speaking with conviction and determination about the anti-aging concept. He has a passion to reverse the signs, symptoms, and ravages of aging. As you listen to him, you come to realize that he has the answers to helping each one of us live a longer and healthier life.

No matter what your age, you have nothing to lose and a healthier, more vital future to gain.

It must be a quirk of human existence that we all abide by a code—why do something today that we can put off until tomorrow? We do this with every aspect of our lives from our finances to our health to our family affairs. Unfortunately when tomorrow comes and goes without any resolution to any of our concerns, we must face the day after.

Start today and join us on a quest for the resolution of challenges to the body, mind, and spirit as we chase the "forever factor."

To learn more about *The Forever Factor*,
visit **www.foreverfactor.com**

Table of Contents

Part One

"Meet James J. Barber, M.D."

"The family is one of nature's masterpieces."
—*George Santayana*

Back to the Beginning

I was born in New Castle, Pennsylvania, a small, very ethnic town about 50 miles north of Pittsburgh. I lived in a lower middle class, very ethnic neighborhood, where everyone looked after and respected each other. It wasn't necessary to lock your doors, because the neighborhood was an extension of your family.

Having the "right" name in our town didn't matter, but having the right nickname did. Some of my friends were called Big Head Elisco, Rabbi Litrenta, Johnny Beans Paolone, and Eugene Tomato Tomelleo. I was known as JB or Doc.

We lived in small houses, sometimes called row houses. No one had a lawn, so we had to play wherever we could find a place. We didn't even have a basketball standard. We just fastened a hoop to a telephone pole and played in the street.

There was an empty field where we played baseball. When someone hit a home run, the ball would go over the fence into old Mr. Cresce's garden. Mr. Cresce had a store, and he would gather up all the home run balls and take them to his store to sell. If you wanted your ball back, you would have to pay Mr. Cresce 50 cents.

We would play hide and seek around the neighborhood. One time little Richard Cumo, we called him "Cub," hid under someone's front porch. While he was waiting for someone to find him, he fell asleep. No one called the police because we all

3

knew he would eventually be located. It took quite a while, but we found him.

In common with the rest of the families in our neighborhood, we didn't have much in the way of worldly goods. However, we didn't realize we were poor, because we had the most important things—the love of our parents and the love of our friends.

Looking back now, even allowing for the mellowing effect of memory, I realize that I had a great life. A key ingredient in making my growing up years so happy was having such a wonderful family.

My grandmother, the matriarch of the family, lived with us. We all called her Mae, since in Italy she would have been known as Mater. All the holidays were built around her. When Christmas came, Aunt Theresa, Uncle Bob, and their family would all come to our house. I remember spending endless hours around the table playing cards, talking about the old country, and discussing the important things of life.

I may not have fully appreciated them at the time, but, reflecting back now after having a child of my own, I realize I had the best parents in the world. My father, James, was English by descent. He had a tough upbringing and lived in several different homes while growing up. He was a tremendously hard-working person, employed by a cement company. During the summers, I would work with him. While some of the guys would sit around waiting for a paycheck, Dad didn't stop. Since I was his son, I had to show Dad's co-workers that I could work hard, too. We would often work without any breaks at all.

I realized that Dad's job was tough and it was putting tremendous stress on his life. To this day, I retain vivid images of Dad coming home after working 12 to 16 hours, with the cement dust literally seeping from his pores. Coughing, he would look absolutely exhausted. I'd watch him and, even though I was a teenager at the time, I knew that he wasn't healthy.

My mother, Carmelita, was a four foot, ten inch, ninety-pound Italian lady who was the foundation of our family, the glue that held us together. She worked all day at a bridal store, hand-making dresses to supplement the family income.

Behind the bridal store, started by my grandmother, there was a little apartment. After school, we would go there and do our homework and have dinner. Our family would gather around the table where we would talk together, sharing the happenings of the day. After dinner, Mother would sit and help my younger sister Laureen, my two younger brothers, Chuck (nicknamed Juice) and Bob (nicknamed Bo), and me with our homework.

My parents were willing to work so hard because they wanted to help their children. Every cent they earned went to us. They never spent a nickel on themselves. My mother wore the same housedress for as long as I can remember, because she didn't want to spend money on anything except her children. My parents invested everything back into our family in order to make life better for us.

This upbringing proved to be a firm foundation for my life, providing me with valuable life lessons:

A Sense of Industry—My upbringing gave me a basis for wanting to be a better person. I was taught to work hard for what I needed, and to be willing to sacrifice for the important things.

A Sense of Purpose—In those days a sense of purpose was part of our lives. I understood life wasn't to be wasted. Life was not only to be enjoyed, but it should also be fulfilling. It was important to give something back—to make a difference for those that follow.

A Sense of Values—My mother imparted to us her values. She taught us to always remember family and to always remember God. She discussed the important things of life with her children, and emphasized the value of living. She'd look at me and say, "Live! Just be happy."

A Sense of Self—My upbringing set the foundation for the rest of my life. From my roots, I gained a sense of self and the determination to accomplish my mission in life. I always wanted to succeed and never let my parents down.

Family, values, and purpose anchored my life at an early age. In essence, I determined that what I desired most was to realize my mother's admonition to "Live! And be happy," and to help others do so as well.

*"We are here to add what we can to life,
not to get what we can from it."*
—*William Osler*

Selecting a Course

As the oldest child in the family, I was the first one in my family to have the opportunity to go to college. I wanted to do well, and I took school very seriously. I attended the University of Pittsburgh where I obtained my Bachelor of Science degree. After graduating from medical school three years later, I completed my internship and residency in surgery at Cedars Sinai Medical Center in Los Angeles, California. Following my residency, I attended the Texas Medical Center in Houston to become a plastic surgeon.

Looking back, I guess I always wanted to be a doctor. Even as a child, I was fascinated with the human body and how we develop perfectly as organisms. I was constantly reading books about the human body and how it worked.

There were other things, however, that influenced my decision to become a physician. There were life experiences that helped steer me in the direction of medicine.

My first fishing trip when I was about seven years old had a great impact on me. My brother Bo and I were standing on the river bank, and Dad had moved upstream from us. Bo wandered too close to the edge, fell in the river, and was immediately swept downstream. I still remember the helplessness and hopelessness I felt at that moment watching my little brother. Young as I was, I realized that he was in trouble and something terrible could happen to him. Just as I took a deep

7

breath to yell for help, I witnessed a miracle. A man by the name of Richard Houston happened to be around the bend just as Bo was being swept into the rapids. Richard jumped in and saved Bo's life. This episode had a terrific influence on me because, even though I was just a child, I understood the value of life and realized how quickly it could end, snuffed out, the vitality and the youthfulness ended. This fired in me the desire to help prolong life—to follow in Richard Houston's footsteps and be a miracle worker for someone else.

I also had family influences on my decision to become a doctor. My uncle, Robert Cassella, was a physician. Sitting around the dinner table growing up, I remember listening to Uncle Bob share stories about being a doctor. I really admired my uncle and the work he accomplished through medicine. I wanted to follow in his footsteps.

The incident that really sealed my decision to become a doctor, specializing in plastic surgery, was an accident I had while playing summer league baseball my senior year at the University of Pittsburgh. I was hit in the face by a batted ball, and the bones surrounding my right cheek were broken.

I will never forget looking in the mirror after the accident. The boney cavity containing my eyeball and its associated muscles, nerves, and vessels had been fractured, and my eyeball had dropped down into the area of the socket. I still remember how I felt as I viewed my disfigured face. It was swollen, black and blue, and, to me, looked monstrous.

Forever etched in my memory is the transformation that my plastic surgeon, Dr. Dwight Hanna, was able to do for me. He used his scalpel, talent, and medical expertise to transform a hideous, unrecognizable face back into mine. Through surgery, Dr. Hanna literally erased the damage to my face. I was mesmerized and grateful as I witnessed the gift my plastic surgeon had given me.

After having that surgery, it was an easy decision to go to medical school. I had glimpsed the healing powers of plastic surgery firsthand. I realized that this could be a tool to not only help someone feel better about themselves; but, in reconstructive surgery, to help those who had been maimed or born with birth defects to become anatomically normal. I began to study and to apply to medical schools. I was going to become a plastic surgeon!

When I began my medical training, I had numerous life-changing experiences. I will always remember the first time I delivered a baby as a medical student. It was the most miraculous thing I had ever seen. I was thrilled to be allowed to participate in this miracle, to assist in the delivery of a new life, and to share in the joy and happiness of the family.

On the other hand, I also remember experiencing death for the first time as a doctor. I was a resident, working with a team to try and save a four-year-old girl who had been in a terrible motor vehicle accident. We tried to resuscitate her for what seemed like hours and hours. Finally, we had to recognize the futility of our efforts and realize that we couldn't save her. It was difficult to hold back the tears as I stood there, watching the life draining away from this beautiful young child who had so much to live for—so much to give. I was once again reminded of how precious the gift of human life is.

There are a myriad of procedures to go through in becoming a plastic surgeon. I first trained in Beverly Hills at Cedars Sinai Medical Center. There I saw some of the biggest stars in the world who were sick and receiving treatment. I came to realize that although these people had the best the world had to offer—money, fame, beautiful mansions, and expensive cars—this didn't insulate them from the illness and suffering of everyday life.

This put life into perspective for me. I realized that rich and poor alike experience illness and suffering. Consequently, rich and poor alike should have access to the benefits of medicine and science to make life better. I began to think how great it would be to extend and improve human life for everyone—to help all people lead healthier, more productive lives.

After Cedars Sinai, I went on to Texas Medical Center in Houston to continue my medical training. There I saw everything from an individual mangled by a lion to a man whose face was crushed when he fell off an oil derrick.

I worked with patients who had severed arms or fingers, requiring replantation of the limbs or digits. One of these patients stands out the most. He was a musician and found tremendous joy in playing the piano. He returned to thank us for restoring his fingers, and his gratitude was heartfelt and humbling to me.

In Houston, one of the most horrific cases I experienced was that of a 13-year-old boy who had grabbed a high tension wire. He received 2nd and 3rd degree burns covering 70 percent of his body. I looked at this young boy who was in so much pain, wondering if his life would be worth living. He did survive, and over the next two years he underwent many surgeries.

However, even after numerous skin grafts and other surgical treatments had been performed, he still couldn't be classified as normal. Despite this, I remember him looking up at us—with deformities, scars and his eyelids singed away—to simply say, "Thank you for saving my life." This experience underlined the realization that human life is the most precious gift we have.

This concept was reinforced for me when, during my residency program, I traveled to the Philippines with a group of plastic surgeons to operate on people who otherwise couldn't afford treatment. It is hard to adequately describe the poverty, squalor, and immense amount of deformity we saw there.

My heart was touched by the parents who would bring their little ones who had been born with cleft lips, cleft palates, and birth defects. The people would bring us chickens or pigs—the only material things they owned—to offer as payment for medical services for their children. These parents wanted nothing more than to help their children have healthy, normal lives.

My experience in the Philippines was a very moving one. It affirmed that being a plastic surgeon was what I truly wanted. I now saw plastic surgery as an opportunity to aid and ease the burden of mankind. By being a plastic surgeon, I could perform cosmetic procedures to help people feel better about themselves, and I could also use my skill to bring relief and joy into the lives of those with birth defects, burns, or crippling deformities. Few things bring more satisfaction to a physician than to know he could give another human being a better quality of life, to help them better function in the world, to feel their worth, to recognize their capabilities, and to become an asset to society.

After leaving Houston and going back to California for additional training, I returned to Pittsburgh to open my practice. This was my home and I wanted to be near my parents and give something back to them for sacrificing so much for me.

In the process of becoming a doctor, I had witnessed all kinds of suffering and gained a new perspective on life. People used to tell me that being sick or being old is only a state of mind. I couldn't tell that to somebody with diabetes, completely bed-ridden, who was losing their toes or feet. I couldn't tell that to people who had suffered strokes and couldn't talk. I couldn't tell them it was only in their minds. But, even as I grasped the realities of illness, I understood some situations could be prevented or improved.

Some of the most jubilant feelings I have experienced as a doctor are when I am in a position to tell someone that they are cancer free, and that they are going to be able to live a normal life. I share the joy and relief a patient feels when they look at their children and grandchildren and realize they still have the gift of time to share with their loved ones. They still have an opportunity to be an influence for good in others' lives.

Conversely, the most dejection I have ever felt is when I have had to tell someone that there was no hope—that there is nothing that can be done to save them. Doctors, with our medical knowledge, like to think of ourselves as being able to do anything. However, when faced with a hopeless situation, we realize just how limited we really are. During these times we are reminded that there is only so much God allows us to do.

In returning to Pittsburgh to set up my own plastic surgery practice, I was soon to experience that reality personally.

"Destiny is no matter of chance. It is a matter of choice. It is not a thing to be waited for, it is a thing to be achieved."
—*William Jennings Bryan*

Finding a Focus

I had been practicing as a young surgeon in Pittsburgh for only about nine months when I got a call from Dr. Jim Bowers, my mother's physician. He said, "Jim, I have some bad news for you. Your mother has pneumonia."

I was surprised by this news because I had just seen her a few days earlier. Dr. Bowers then told me that Mother had broken ribs. I was shocked and immediately asked if she had been in an accident. Dr. Bowers replied, "No, she's been sick for a while. She's been walking around with six broken ribs for the last couple of weeks. She didn't tell anybody, because she didn't want everybody to worry. Jim, your mother has Plasma Cell Myeloma. She doesn't have long to live—maybe three to six months."

The first thing I ever bought for myself was a watch. Although it was brand new, the watch stopped working at the exact time that I was told my mother was terminal, and it never worked again.

I was determined to get my mother the best medical help available. I took her to the Mayo clinic and M.D. Anderson Hospital. I also set up appointments for her with specialists all over the country to see if there was anything that could be done, but each time the answer was the same. My mother had a terminal illness, she was going to die, and there was nothing that could be done to prevent it.

When I had opened my own practice, I bought my mother an emerald ring. She had always wanted one, and she had teased me that someday when I was a doctor I would buy one for her. On her death bed, my mother took that ring off, gave it to my father, and told him to take care of it. I knew at that moment she had given up. She looked at her family gathered around her and, with her last breath told us, "Love God, love each other, live and be happy."

My life was jolted by the death of my mother, and I was nagged by questions. She was only 58 years old! I asked myself, "How could someone who is only 58 years old die when others can live to be a 110 or 120? What made my mother different from those with greater longevity?" I had to find out! I wanted—I needed answers.

I began to study anti-aging, and came up with even more questions: What is really the method by which we age? Is aging a disease process? Do diet, nutrition, or air pollutants affect aging? Do our habits and the way we handle ourselves make a difference? What makes us age faster than other people?

I continued to search for an answer. Then a few years ago outside of New York City I came together with a group of 25 other physicians. We formed a group called Longevity Institute International. We met together to pool our efforts and develop solutions to overcome disease and disability. We also sought to discover ways to promote being healthy for as long as possible, and to find ways of prolonging life.

It was the first time there was a blending of medical science with medical technology to ascertain how we age. Out of that meeting, I found answers and came up with a new focus for my practice of medicine.

"A man is not old as long as he is seeking something."
—*Jean Rostand*

Four Basic Theories of Aging

Out of The Longevity Institute International meetings, we discovered that there are four basic theories of aging. Those four theories are:

The Free Radical
The Wear and Tear
The Neuroendocrine
Genetic

THE FREE RADICAL THEORY OF AGING

The Free Radical Theory of Aging states that every time you consume something, you generate what is called *Free Radicals*. There is a structure in the cell called the mitochondrion, which is a powerhouse to the cell. When you take in food sources, the mitochondrion generates energy and, as a by-product, it gives off an oxygen ion with a negative charge that is called a *free radical*.

This free radical is a scavenger. It looks around and says, "I need another electron to make me free—to make me not so agitated. I'm going to bombard the muscle cells and cause atrophy. I'm going to bombard the brain cells and cause such things as Parkinson's Disease and Alzheimer's. I'm going to bombard the spleen and decrease the immune system."

In essence, free radicals are powerful elements that

bombard the cell membranes. When these membranes get holes poked in them, the fat in the cell membrane becomes rancid and builds up toxins in our bodies.

Free radicals also damage the sites where hormones are located and bound to the cell. Hormones are a product of living cells that circulate in body fluids and have a specific affect on the activity of cells remote from their point of origin.

Hormones are important because they link to certain parts on the cell membrane and perform a lock and key mechanism, which turns on the functions of the cell. Over time, the free radicals damage those sites, so that the lock and key no longer work. The result is that even though hormones are still being produced, they have become less effective.

The body fights back, refusing to just give in to the barrage of free radical assaults. It recognizes the need for fortification and calls upon the enzymes and other chemicals called antioxidants. Then the war is on between the robbers of the body—the free radicals—and the antioxidant police force.

Antioxidants are one of the major weapons against free radical aging. They give up electrons to free radicals, so that the free radical can't damage us. The human body has trillions and trillions of cells. Each one of those is bombarded about 10,000 times a day by free radicals. Since this bombardment occurs day after day after day, over the course of time, it damages the cells and the DNA so much that it turns on those genes which cause us to age and to develop diseases associated with aging, such as diabetes and arthritis.

Dr. Lester Packer, Ph.D, a world renowned scientist from the University of California, Berkeley, has a revolutionary theory concerning antioxidants. Dr. Packer, dubbed by his colleagues "Dr. Antioxidant," has dedicated nearly five decades of research into the biochemistry of antioxidants. He proposes that antioxidants work in the body not singly but as a network, and that "the sum is greater than its parts." He believes that antioxidants synergize with and greatly enhance the power of each other and, even more importantly, recycle each other.

For instance, Dr. Packer affirms that Coenzyme Q10 enhances the action of vitamin E, that some of the effects ascribed to Co-Q10 are due primarily to its potentiation of vitamin E. Dr. Packer reiterates that it is very difficult to study the effects of a single antioxidant because the whole network is affected, and it is the whole network that produces the manifold results that we see.

Dr. Packer describes network antioxidants as a mutually recycling "juggernaut" against the lethal forces of oxidation. He shows this particularly in regard to the 5 pivotal antioxidants that he calls "network antioxidants": lipoic acid, coenzyme Q10, vitamin C, vitamin E (all natural varieties of it, not just alpha topopherol), and glutathione.

Lipoic Acid

Lipoic acid is naturally produced in the body, but, as we age, we stop producing it in sufficient quantities. Dr. Packer discovered that lipoic acid differs from other antioxidants in several important ways. First, unlike other antioxidants that have a specific job in the body, lipoic acid is so versatile that it can serve as a "free agent" and pinch hit for the other antioxidants when they are in short supply. It also greatly enhances the potency of vitamins C and E. When combined with lipoic acid, we can see these two antioxidants are more powerful and their beneficial effects more long-lasting than when they stand alone. More proof of this antioxidant's flexibility is its important function of normalizing blood sugar levels.

Coenzyme Q10 (Co-Q10)

Coenzyme Q10 is essential to the body's energy extraction

mechanism. Much like spark plugs are needed to jump-start an engine, Co-Q10 provides the "spark" which starts the mitochondria engines, without which cell life, and thus human life, would cease to exist. Co-Q10 is an antioxidant similar to vitamin E, protecting fat molecules from becoming oxidized or infused with free radicals that go on rampages and irreparably damage cells.

Studies have shown Co-Q10 can increase stamina and reduce angina (chest pain) in heart patients undergoing an exercise treadmill test. This is extremely important, inasmuch as exercise is one of the most effective treatments for heart disease.

Large doses of Co-Q10 have proven highly effective in treating some cases of advanced cancer. When the body has adequate energy, every organ and system can perform well, and the body is more able to fight disease and heal itself.

Vitamin C

If you want to live longer, eat lots of fruits and vegetables and take vitamin C pills, starting now! "A 35-year-old man who eats vitamin C—rich foods and takes vitamin C supplements will slash his chances of heart disease death by two-thirds and live 6.3 years longer," predicts Dr. James Endstrom, UCLA researcher.

In her book, *Stop Aging Now*, Jean Carper states some alarming facts:

- One-fourth of Americans do not get even the minimal rock-bottom daily amount of 60 milligrams of vitamin C that cells need to perform basic biological functions.

- Only 9 percent of Americans eat five daily servings of fruits and vegetables (200-300 milligrams of vitamin C) as urged by the National Cancer Institute.

- According to one study, about 20 percent of healthy older people and 68 percent of elderly nonhospitalized patients had white blood cells deficient in vitamin C.

Overwhelmingly, some 120 studies identify vitamin C as a form of vaccination against cancer. According to Gladys Block, Ph.D., cancer epidemiologist at the University of California, Berkeley, five daily servings of fruits and vegetables contain 200 to 300 milligrams of vitamin C—enough to help retard cancer. But for extra cancer insurance, she suggests you need a supplement. Dr. Block personally takes 2,000 to 3,000 milligrams of vitamin C a day.

Vitamin C, necessary for the production of new cells and tissue, also offers protection of arteries. Surprisingly, modest amounts of vitamin C can drive up good-type HDL (high density lipoproteins) cholesterol that discourages artery clogging. It also reduces bad-type LDL (low density lipoproteins) cholesterol that destroys arteries.

Vitamin C also lowers high blood pressure, strengthens blood vessel walls, makes blood less sticky, and thwarts cholesterol-inspired changes leading to clogged arteries.

In 1970, Dr. Linus Pauling's book, *Vitamin C and the Common Cold*, rocked the medical establishment by suggesting that high doses of vitamin C could shorten the length and severity of a cold. We now know that Vitamin C relieves the symptoms of a cold by reducing the histamine level in the blood stream. Histamines are what cause the runny nose and watery eyes, typical of colds. Taking 250–2,000 milligrams of vitamin C per day is suggested for best results.

Vitamin E

Recently, two new important studies have shown that high doses of vitamin E could strengthen immune function in older people and slow the progression of Alzheimer's disease more effectively than drugs. Vitamin E can also reduce the risk of heart disease and is used as a treatment for hot flashes during menopause.

Vitamin E fights our greatest aging fear, atherosclerosis, the gradual clogging and hardening of arteries that begins in youth, worsens in middle age, and kills about half a million Americans a year, primarily in old age. Atherosclerosis occurs in large part because bad-type LDL blood cholesterol is chemically altered, oxidized or turned rancid and toxic by free radical attacks. If such LDL oxidation does not occur, LDL cholesterol is not able to infiltrate artery walls, which is the first step to stopping plaque buildup and clogging, narrowing, and disintegration of the arteries. Stopping LDL oxidation is what vitamin E supplements do expertly—far better than any other antioxidant vitamin.

Remember, you need at least 100 IU of vitamin E daily to get any measurable protection against heart attacks. Vitamin E, not only rejuvenates old arteries, it also rejuvenates immunity, thwarts cancer, relieves arthritis, postpones cataracts, retards overall blood and brain aging. (*Inasmuch as vitamin E is a natural blood thinner, if you are taking medication to thin your blood, do not take vitamin E supplements without first consulting your physician.*)

Glutathione

You must get your levels of glutathione up if you want to keep your youth and live longer. High blood levels of glutathione predict a long life and good health. Low levels predict early disease and death.

Glutathione, one of the most fascinating antioxidants, is a naturally occurring amino acid in your diet and is also produced by your cells internally as part of the body's magnificently designed detoxification system to fend off free radical damage. Glutathione is the most powerful, versatile, and important of these self-generated antioxidants. "It is the master antioxidant," proclaims John T. Pinto of Memorial Sloan Kettering Cancer Center in New York. Glutathione is the body's main powerhouse for defusing and disposing of free radicals that bring on the woes of aging. It protects every cell, tissue and organ in the body. "If you deplete glutathione, the cell disintegrates and loses its immune activity. If you add glutathione to that ailing cell, it regenerates and becomes immuno-efficient," states Dr. Mara Julius, University of Michigan.

THE WEAR AND TEAR THEORY OF AGING

The Wear and Tear Theory of Aging is easy to understand. Simply put, when you are 20 to 25 years old you can go out, eat hot dogs with chili *and* onions, digest everything, and sleep peacefully all night. However, eat that same cuisine when you get to be 40 to 50 years old, and that hot dog, chili, *and* onions will keep you painfully up for half the night.

The body does its best with what we put in our mouths. However, as we grow older, our body chemistry changes. It becomes more difficult for us to assimilate the nutrients that we need. As our body chemistry changes, we end up with a series of things happening. Because the stomach can't absorb as it once could, the liver has to give up some enzymes. The liver then borrows enzymes from the gall bladder. Because the gall bladder is overworking in a way it shouldn't, it has to borrow from the bones, causing osteoporosis because of calcium depletion. The body ends up overusing and working overtime in a way it wasn't meant to do, accelerating the aging process.

Taking vitamins and\or supplements to ease the overuse and overworking of your body is one way to upset the Wear and

Tear Theory of Aging. However, this is an area where a little bit of knowledge can be a dangerous thing. Anytime you take vitamins or supplements, you must make sure they are in a form that your body can use.

It has been said that Americans have the most expensive urine in the world. Why? Because many end up going to a health food or grocery store looking for "something" beneficial. They seek advice from a 20-year-old clerk, who knows absolutely nothing about vitamins and supplements, who suggests, "Well, everybody is taking X, Y, & Z. I don't know exactly what these products do, but we sure sell a lot of them. Everybody seems to love them."

Those who accept such health advice from a 20-year-old clerk will purchase a variety of products they feel will do the job and that they are sure to love. The problem comes, however, with blending vitamins and supplements in a way you shouldn't, such as taking one product that is incompatible with another, or taking too many products altogether.

For example, those that take water-soluble vitamins have a problem with absorption. Such vitamins are lost quickly after a trip to the bathroom, thereby producing the most expensive urine in the world and effecting little good.

Another area where people get into trouble is using a product they've heard about or seen advertised, without understanding the far-reaching effects of long-term usage. For instance, there are numerous ads on TV for taking products to help you sleep. It is true that these substances will aid with falling asleep. However, it is possible to overdose on or become addicted to some of these products.

The only way to upset the Wear and Tear Theory of Aging is to understand what you should be taking, and when and how you should be taking it. Vitamins, minerals, and supplements have to be in a form that the body can absorb. For example, everyone needs the trace metals, such as zinc and copper, in our body to help us function. If you take a metallic form of these when you are under the age of 30 or 40, you can absorb about 10 percent of them. Taking the same form of trace metals after you get older will result in an absorption rate of only two to three percent. It can't be emphasized enough that vitamins, minerals, and supplements will only make a difference to your aging if you take them in *a form your body can absorb and utilize.*

THE NEUROENDOCRINE THEORY OF AGING

This third theory of aging is one that has been known about for a long time, but has recently been revolutionized. The Neuroendocrine theory says as we get older, our production of many hormones, such as sex and energy hormones, is significantly reduced. In addition, growth hormone, a peptide secreted by the anterior pituitary, is also greatly affected.

The pituitary gland is the master gland of the body. It forms thyroid hormone and adrenocorticotropic hormone. Thyroid hormone is a metabolic regulator in the body. We are talking about thyroid hormone when we refer to regulating the metabolic rate. Adrenocorticotropic hormone acts on the adrenal gland regulating fluid balance and also affects the sex hormones, testosterone and estrogen.

One of the hormones that really affect our lives is growth hormone. Growth hormone is a production of the anterior pituitary and affects everything in the body. After it is secreted, it passes from the pituitary to the liver, changing to insulin growth factor one (IGF-1). IGF-1 factor goes all over the body to reverse some of the first signs and symptoms we see in aging. It affects brain cells, hair color, and even cellulite.

The critical aspect of growth hormone is that beyond the ages of 20—25 it decreases every decade about 14 percent.

Consequently, every decade thereafter, there is a continual reduction in energy and stamina levels, affecting the body's ability to fight the aging process. With aging, there is not only a decrease of growth hormone, but there is also an increase in the production of a substance called somatostatin, which is a blocker to growth hormone. In order to block somatostatin, we can add an amino acid called arginine, which actually takes away the blocker and allows the production of your own growth hormone to be more effective.

Once, growth hormone shots were the only available source to help boost our supply of human growth hormone, also known as HGH. These shots were not only expensive, but could have some serious side affects if used unwisely. Recently a new host of all natural stimulants to growth hormone have been added to the anti-aging regimen. These new products work in a natural and safe manner to help fight the Neuroendocrine decline of our advancing years.

HGH is the ultimate anti-aging therapy. It affects almost every cell in the body, rejuvenating the skin and bones, regenerating the heart, liver, lungs, and kidneys, bringing organ and tissue function back to youthful levels. It is an anti-disease medicine that revitalizes the immune system, lowers the risk factors for heart attack and stroke, improves oxygen uptake in emphysema patients, and prevents osteoporosis. It is under investigation for a host of different diseases from osteoporosis to post-polio syndrome to AIDS.

It is the most effective anti-obesity drug ever discovered, revving up the metabolism to youthful levels, resculpting the body by selectively reducing the fat in the waist, abdomen, hips and thighs, and at the same time increasing muscle mass. It may be plastic surgery in a bottle, smoothing out facial wrinkles; restoring the elasticity, thickness, and contours of youthful skin.

The list of benefits seems to grow with each new study. According to Dr. Ronald Klatz in his book *Grow Young with HGH*, the benefits of growth hormone now include:

• 8.8 percent increase in muscle mass on average after six months without exercise

• 14.4 percent loss of fat on average after six months without dieting

• Higher energy levels

• Enhanced sexual performance

• Regrowth of heart, liver, spleen, kidneys, and other organs that shrink with age

• Greater cardiac output

• Superior immune function

• Increased exercise performance

• Better kidney function

• Lowered blood pressure

• Improved cholesterol profile, with higher HDL and lower LDL

• Stronger Bones

• Faster wound healing

• Younger, tighter, thicker skin

• Hair regrowth

• Wrinkle removal

• Elimination of cellulite

• Sharper vision

• Mood elevation

• Increased memory retention

• Improved sleep

Human Growth Hormone Levels As Related to Aging

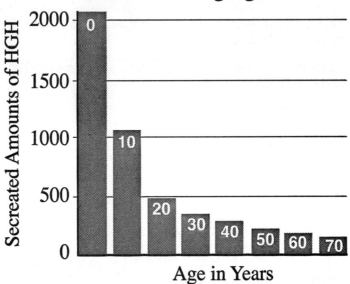

LOOK AT THE AMAZING TEST RESULTS

Results from a study [effects of Growth Hormone administration 202 patients age 39-74] by L. Casserry M.D., Ph.D. and Edmund Chein M.D., Medical College of Wisconsin and Palm Springs Life

Body Fat Loss	82% Improvement
Wrinkle Reduction	61% Improvement
Energy Level	84% Improvement
Muscle Strength	88% Improvement
Sexual Potency	75% Improvement
Emotional Stability	67% Improvement
Memory	62% Improvement

GENETIC THEORY OF AGING

The Genetic Theory of Aging is currently on the cutting edge of science. The mapping of the human genome is going to be the greatest breakthrough in the history of medicine. It is going to do for medicine what the industrial revolution did for the productions of goods in the early part of the century. The Human Genome Project, sponsored in the United States by the Department of Energy and National Institutes of Health, has created the field of genomics, which has allowed us to understand genetic material on a large scale. The medical industry is building upon this genetic knowledge, using resources and technologies emanating from the Human Genome Project, to further our understanding of genetic contributions to human health. Genetics is playing an increasingly important role in the diagnosis, monitoring, and treatment of diseases.

The long-range goal is to use this genetic information to develop new ways to treat, cure, or even prevent the thousands of diseases that afflict humankind. Drug design will be revolutionized as researchers create new classes of medicines based on a reasoned approach using gene sequence and protein structure function information, rather than the traditional trial-and-error method. Because of the genetic approach, these projected drugs promise to have fewer side effects than many of today's current medicines.

The ultimate goal of genome research is to find all the genes in the DNA sequence and to develop tools for using this information in the study of human biology and medicine. With the mapping of the human genome, we are actually able to get to the DNA level. This will not only allow us to study why Parkinson's, Alzheimer's, diabetes, cancer, and other diseases occur, but will also give us the means of altering the DNA in such a way so that we can prevent those diseases from happening. In essence, when the types of diseases listed above are eradicated, human life will be extended astronomically.

It's only when DNA goes out of whack that we start seeing the development of disease and painful ailments. When you are young, you are producing DNA, your cells are dividing, and you are healthy. When there are DNA problems and your cells change just a little bit; you have the onset of health problems, such as diabetes and arthritis.

The body turns against itself because the DNA code is damaged. We can now foresee being able to repair that DNA. Growth hormones are already being used to facilitate the influx of proteins, nucleic acids, and amino acids into the internal portion of the cell nucleus to help it repair itself.

The big breakthrough we are going to see, however, is in the substance called telomerase. Telomerase is a substance which controls cell divisions. Every cell in the body is programmed for roughly 70 cell divisions. As the body ages and the cell approaches what is known as the Hayflick limit, which is the maximum number of times the cell can divide, the aging gene is ignited and programs cell death or apoptosis.

This is similar to the oil light going on in your car. If the oil light comes on, it tells the driver that oil needs to be added. If no oil is added to your engine, it will overheat and, eventually, grind to a screeching halt. The same thing is true with the cells in your body. The age light goes on and tells the cell, "You are going to start aging."

Research is now focusing on the X-like structure called the telomere that contains the DNA bases with the genetic code of the body. Upon each cell division, a sheath that protects the DNA shortens. As it does this, the DNA bases, which were once protected, are now exposed. This allows the DNA to be attacked by chemicals in the air, as well as toxins and free radicals in the body, damaging the DNA and depositing it as "garbage." When this garbage accumulates, it kicks on the body's age light, the aging gene, that tells the body it's time for apoptosis, or in other words, time to die.

Telomerase, a substance that acts at the level of the telomere, is a key in extending healthy aging. The research on the Genetic Theory of Aging is in fooling the sheath on the telomere into shortening not on every cell division but instead on shortening on every second or third cell division, therefore extending the lifespan of the cell and ultimately the organism to lengths previously only imagined—healthy, vital, productive years free of disease and disability.

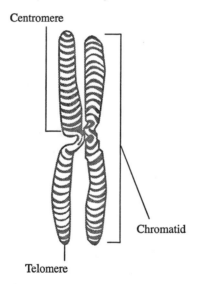

Centromere

Chromatid

Telomere

Telomerase acts upon the chromosome at a
site known as the telomere

Other cutting edge research is focusing on the use of substances such as L-Carnosine. Carnosine is a combination of amino acids, alanine and histidine. This combination in the form of Carnosine has been shown to break glycation end products. Products of glucose and protein cause such debilitating states as cataracts and amyloidosis. Researchers in Russia and

Australia have used eye drops of N-acetyl Carnosine to eradicate cataracts. In fact, studies in vivo, which is at the cellular level, have shown L-Carnosine to increase cell division by 25 percent and to increase cell longevity by an astounding 300 percent.

At the time of Julius Caesar, the average life expectancy was 25 years old. At the turn of the 20th century, it was 47 years old. Now, life expectancy is between 75 to 77 years old. There are approximately 70,000 people in the United States today who are around 100 years old. By the year 2050, due to genomic research, scientists foresee between 2.4 and 4 million people living beyond the age of 100.

Other noted researchers and anti-aging experts, such as Brian Larsen of Orem, Utah, have attacked the genetic theory of aging from a revolutionary standpoint, the elemental level of the DNA. This research focuses on carrier processes that repair DNA and, in effect, alter mistakes in the genetic code, thereby improving and, in many cases, relieving the debilitating diseases of aging.

This is just some of the information and technology that came out of The Longevity Institute International meetings. The other physicians and I that form this group realize that we are in the midst of a miraculous break-through in anti-aging/longevity medicine. Scientific information regarding anti-aging/longevity is doubling every 2.7 to 3 years. That not only means that what we know today will be outmoded in 3 years, it also means that viable scientific knowledge in this field will be doubled in that same time period.

I am committed to strengthening ties with anti-aging medicine and remaining on the forefront of anti-aging research developments. I am determined to find ways to use the scientific breakthroughs discussed above to succeed in the search of the "forever factor."

"Age does not depend upon years, but upon temperament and health."
—Tyron Edwards

Developing a Philosophy

Even before Ponce de Leon searched for the "Fountain of Youth," man has been intrigued by the notion of immortality—of eternal youth. When I became involved with the Longevity Institute International, I did not find the "Fountain of Youth," but I did discover hope. I found research-based answers, practical theory, and cutting-edge technology, all useful weapons in the anti-aging war.

As I researched and studied anti-aging, I discovered that this branch of medicine was a natural match with plastic surgery. I can reverse aging by doing a face lift or someone's eyelids and make them look younger. But, that alone will not free them from the trap of old age. Cosmetic surgery on the outside needs to be coupled with changes on the inside to promote health and longevity. Without changing the inside, a cosmetic surgery patient will return in five or six years with wrinkles back and tummy tucks stretched. I realize that by incorporating anti-aging medicine into plastic surgery techniques I can treat the whole patient.

I am also cognizant of the universal value of anti-aging medicine. I know that everyone needs freedom from the negative effects of aging, from becoming decrepit, frail, senile, and physically broken-down. I understand that anti-aging medicine has tools to help everyone fight the disease of aging.

One such useful tool I discovered is age scans. Age scans

are tests to compare the two ways people age, chronologically and biologically. Age changes affect different parts of the body at different times. These age changes occur in the DNA, tissues, organs, and hormone levels, along with every component of the human body. Chronological age measures the amount of time that has gone by since birth. Biological age measures the age range at which we function. For example, there might be a man who is chronologically 65, but, biologically, looks and moves like a 45-year-old; or, there might be a woman who is chronologically 80, but, biologically, has the mental acuity of a 60-year-old. Biological age differs dramatically from individual to individual.

Age scans test such areas as respiratory performance, vibratory sensation, and cognitive functioning. The results of the age scan are compared to a "norm" to determine biological versus chronological age.

A good friend of mine, Rick Gradisek, a 42-year-old dentist in Pittsburgh, tested out on the age scan as being biologically 52 years old. This indicated to me that Rick was aging much quicker than he should due to free radical damage. I placed Rick on a regimen of antioxidants and growth hormones, and retested him approximately 6 months later. At that time, I discovered Rick had reversed his biological age to 39.

I am also impressed with the application of DNA testing in fighting aging. We can test up to a 150 enzyme panel of DNA, break down the DNA, and examine all the constituents. It is extremely useful and important to recognize some of the basic markers and risk factors for premature aging. This allows us to pinpoint areas where anti-aging measures can make a difference.

As I have studied anti-aging, I have become aware of anti-aging field research on population pockets around the world where people routinely live to be 110 to 120, enjoying good health throughout their lifetimes. Different factors of life and products native to these areas are being examined to test their efficacy in promoting good health and longevity. Products such as Noni, Aloe Vera, Peruvian Maca, and Guggul are just a few of the offshoots of these intensive studies.

I have been galvanized as a physician to have anti-aging research and technology available to assist in my plastic surgery practice, and have been impressed by the results I've observed in patients from anti-aging applications. After the death of my mother, I set out to seek answers to aging. However, I never intended the results of my search to be limited to my practice.

I have been filled with an intense desire to help as many people as possible benefit from the advantages of anti-aging medicine. I have continued to research, brainstorm, and seek answers. I have consulted with experts in their fields to seek ways individuals could help themselves with aging, and even reverse the effects of aging.

The end product of my consultations, medical studies, field research, scientific brainstorming, personal upbringing, and familial influence has been the realization that what would be most helpful to anyone in the battle against aging is to adopt an anti-aging philosophy of life.

If people could catch the vision of anti-aging possibilities, have the courage to examine their lifestyles, attitudes, and mind-sets, and have the resolution to make needed changes, they could live longer and better.

The resulting chapters are the various facets of my anti-aging philosophy of life. Each of us can begin our own personal search to find the "forever factor" to help us overcome the difficulties of aging today. The "Fountain of Youth" does not exist. There is no magical cure-all. There are, however, answers to aging. There are changes we can make, steps we can take, and research we can learn from in order to become as healthy as it is possible for us to be. In the words of Henry James, "It is time for us to start living the life we imagined."

Part Two

"Armed Against Aging"

I believe it's important to be aware of the health strategies that support anti-aging. By applying the principles that are discussed in Part Two, you can better arm yourself to fight the aging battle.

"Glutton: one who digs his grave with his teeth."
—*French Proverb*

"An Apple a Day . . ."

In the movie *The Dead Poets Society*, the central character is a gifted, concerned teacher, who is trying to inspire his students with the courage to go after their dreams, to be true to themselves, and to become the best that they can be. Throughout the movie, we hear the phrase "carpe diem," which means, "seize the day," or, in other words, *make the most of today—don't procrastinate, don't hesitate, don't wait until tomorrow.*

As a physician, I probably have a little different take on that phrase because most of the patients I see live by the philosophy "carpe cras," meaning "seize tomorrow." Case in point: picture a man sitting on a couch, snacking from a bag of Doritos, a Snickers candy bar, and a package of Ho-Ho's, while he sips a Diet Coke. He apparently fantasizes that drinking the Diet Coke will eradicate all the empty calories he is consuming from the Doritos, Snickers, and Ho-Ho's. In actual fact, what he's saying to himself is, "Tomorrow I'll start eating better, and cut out all the junk food." That philosophy is "carpe cras" thinking. Tomorrow, he will have three cans of Diet Coke, a couple of pastrami sandwiches, chips, and a large slice of apple pie—and that's only lunch. He consoles himself with the thought that when he has time to make a run to the grocery store and pick up some healthier food, he'll change his eating habits. The problem, of course, is that tomorrow never comes. In the meantime, the overeating and poor nutrition take their toll, damaging the body and hastening the aging process.

The temptation to eat poorly comes from many sources. Every fast food advertised on TV is calculated to look delicious, mouth-watering, and readily available just around the corner. At sporting events, we are enticed with hot dogs, hamburgers, cheese-smothered nachos, and fresh peanuts. Movie complexes, before allowing us to enter the theater, direct us past the concession stand, where we are tantalized with hot popcorn dripping in butter, high calorie drinks, and sugary snacks, all in the extra-large, mega-huge, containing enough calories to feed a family of four, single-serving size.

Being eager consumers, caught up in the moment, entrenched in the "carpe cras" mentality, we seldom remember these things are not good for us, telling ourselves, "I'll eat this now, and start watching what I eat tomorrow." Then the day after tomorrow comes. Were any changes made?

Lifestyles have changed throughout the years, and that has only added further fuel to the poor nutritional fire. The close family relationships with the family sitting down together for the evening meal that I remember and cherish, have, for many, gone by the way-side. Today is the day of convenience products, super-size fast food, and eating on the run. Consequently, more and more Americans are eating larger portions of fatty foods and empty calories, suffering from signs of malnutrition in one of the wealthiest countries in the world.

If each one of us would realistically examine our eating habits *today*, we would probably find some places where positive changes could be made. A good start would be to remember what our grandmothers taught us: "An apple a day keeps the doctor away, eat *all* your vegetables, and milk helps build bones and teeth."

In addition to grandmother's advice, the U.S. Departments of Agriculture and Health and Human Services suggest the following Dietary Guidelines for Americans, which consist of seven basic principals for developing and maintaining a healthier diet. These Guidelines represent the best thinking in the field of nutrition and health today and are the basis for all federal nutrition information and education programs. They emphasize balance, variety, and moderation in the overall diet.

The Dietary Guidelines for Americans are:

Eat a variety of foods
Maintain desirable weight
Avoid too much fat, saturated fat, and cholesterol
Eat foods with adequate starch and fiber
Avoid too much sugar
Avoid too much sodium
If you drink alcoholic beverages, do so in moderation

Preparing foods in the Dietary Guidelines' style doesn't mean eliminating **all** fat, sugars (refers to granulated sugar and other sweeteners such as syrups, honey, and molasses), and sodium; it just means avoiding too much. **Balance is the key!** Balance the foods that tend to be high in fat, sugars, or sodium with other foods that contain less of these components. If you tend to prepare foods that are high in less healthy elements, gradually begin to reduce the amounts of these items. For instance, if you've decided to cut back on fat, sugar, and sodium in your diet, using less of these in food preparation is one important way to reach your goal.

We are all familiar with the fact that it is important to include daily servings from the Four Food Groups:

Fruits and vegetables
Grains and Cereals
Dairy products
Protein

The important reason for eating a variety of foods is to maintain good health. Eating from the four food groups is the easiest way to get adequate nutrition. It is certainly possible to be a vegetarian and still be healthy, but it is usually more difficult to get the proper amount of protein in your diet.

Forty-three million people suffer from arthritis, including 300,000 children. Two million lives are affected by Fibromyalgia. An equally impressive number of "weekend warriors" and everyday athletes face a myriad of joint pains and muscle aches brought on by their attempts to become NBA stars during Saturday afternoon pick-up games. The only figure more staggering than the amount of individuals living with pain is the number of theories on how to alleviate it.

Perhaps surprisingly, the most effective method of combating the types of pain described above is with a complete program of diet, exercise, and supplementation. Everyone, especially those suffering from arthritis, can benefit from a healthy well-balanced diet with plenty of vegetables, fruits, whole grain products and a limited amount of sugar, salt, and saturated fat. Especially important is the amount and ratio of Omega-6 and Omega-3 fatty acids. Omega 6 fatty acids are found largely in flaxseed, with smaller amounts existing in soy and canola. Omega-3 fatty acids are of two types: eicosapentanoic acid (EPA) and docosahexanoic acid (DHA). These do a number of things such as balance cholesterol levels, decrease the risk of heart disease and cancer, and decrease pain and inflammation of joints. Both sources of omega-3 fatty acids are found in fish sources like salmon, tuna, herring, mackerel, and swordfish.

Supplementation, in combination with topical analgesic lotions, can help relieve the suffering of arthritis and attack the aches and pains of muscle and joint problems. Some of these may include glucosamine, chondroitin, omega-3 fatty acids, aloe vera, MSM, vitamins C and E, emu oil, evening primrose oil, boswelia, and tumeric.

Jean Carper, a leading nutrition expert, presents an argument for including fish as a protein in your diet. She encourages, "Eat fish! The case is so compelling that you absolutely must pay attention. . . . Fish's secret is its unique oil (omega-3 fatty acids), which is essential for proper cell functioning."

Carper also points out that most of us get only 15 percent of the omega-3 we need. The latest research on fish oil's life-saving potential relates to the more than 250,000 heart attack deaths which take place every year, half of which have no warning signs. Harvard research suggests eating fatty fish could stop an astonishing 80 percent of such deaths in men, and states that the more women eat fish, the *less likely* they are to have a heart attack or die of a "cardiac event."

You don't even have to consume a lot of fish to reap the benefits. According to research, eating fish only once a week could cut heart attack risk by as much as 29 percent. A week's quota of fish might be equal to 13 oz. of canned salmon or 6 oz. fresh mackerel. Carper reports that fish is also given credit for cutting strokes, blocking cancer development, and stimulating brain function.

CARBOHYDRATES, FATS, AND PROTEINS

All food can be divided into three parts: carbohydrates, fats, and proteins. The first two generate fuel for the body to run on, while the third provides raw materials for development of cells and tissues.

Carbohydrates

Carbohydrates fuel the muscles during exercise and help maintain tissue protein. They also furnish the glucose for the brain and nervous system to run on.

- Carbohydrates have four calories per gram and it takes 100—150 grams of carbohydrates to prevent drawing on the body's protein.

- There are two kinds of carbohydrates, complex and refined.

- Complex carbohydrates are fruits, vegetables, and whole grains. These are considered the good carbohydrates because they convert to blood sugar more slowly and provide energy longer, as well as being excellent sources of vitamins, minerals, and fiber.

- Refined carbohydrates, the black sheep of the carbohydrate family, are just the opposite of complex carbohydrates. They are the things our grandmothers' told us to avoid because they would rot our teeth. Refined carbohydrates include such things as sugars, candy, soft drinks, desserts, etc. They are poor nutritional choices because they have little nutritional value, pack a load of calories, and offer short-term energy jags that are rapidly depleted.

Fats

Fats are a necessary part of our diet, but obviously need to be used in moderation. The following are some facts about fats to keep in mind:

- All fats have nine calories per gram.

- Fats are the main forms in which energy is stored.

- Fats are the energy source for prolonged low-to-moderate intensity exercise.

- Fats are a source of vitamins A, D, E, and K.

- Simple fats are divided into saturated fatty acids and unsaturated fats.

- Saturated fatty acids, which are solid at room temperature, are obtained from animal fats and include meat, egg yolks, dairy products, and shellfish.

- Unsaturated fats, which are liquid at room temperature, come from plant sources, including corn oil, safflower oil, olive oil, and peanut oil.

- Compound fats are simple fats combined with other chemicals. The main groups are phospholipids, a key component of cell membranes, and lipoproteins, which transport fat in the blood. These are the HDLs (high density lipoproteins), LDLs (low density lipoproteins), and VLDL (very low density lipoproteins). The VLDL group is the most unhealthy. They carry fat throughout the body where it can form deposits in the arteries, causing atherosclerosis, also known as narrowing of the arteries.

- Derived fats combine simple and compound fats. The best known of the derived fats is cholesterol. Despite its bad reputation, cholesterol is essential for many bodily functions, including the synthesis of vitamin D and making female sex steroid hormones. The main dietary sources of cholesterol are egg yolks, organ meats, shellfish, and dairy products (not the low or no fat varieties).

Proteins

Proteins are building blocks for the cells and tissues:

- Proteins have four calories per gram.

- Proteins make up one-half of dry body weight, including muscles, skin, bones, hair, teeth, eyes, nails, and scar tissue.

- Hormones and enzymes, which orchestrate all the activities of the body, are proteins.

- Proteins help maintain water, acid, and base balance, confer resistance to disease, carry oxygen in the blood, maintain growth, and repair cells and tissues.
- Amino acids, the building blocks of protein, are broken into two groups, essential and nonessential. Essential amino acids cannot be synthesized by the body and must be supplied from the outside. Low amounts of essential amino acids will stop protein synthesis.
- Proteins comes from animal and plant sources. Animal proteins, such as meat, milk, milk products, fish, poultry, and eggs, contain all the essential amino acids in the correct proportions.
- Plant proteins, such as grains and beans, usually lack one or more essential amino acid, but can be combined to form balanced proteins.
- Excess protein is converted to fat and stored in fat cells.

VITAMINS, MINERALS, FIBER, AND WATER

Vitamins, minerals, fiber, and water are also essential elements of a balanced diet.

<u>Vitamins</u>
- Vitamins are organic substances in foods that are essential in small amounts for body processes.
- Vitamins facilitate energy release from fat, carbohydrates, and protein.
- Vitamins are vital for formulation of red blood cells, connective tissue, proteins, and DNA. Deficiencies cause malnutrition of body processes.
- Fat-soluble vitamins, A, D, E, and K, are stored in body fat and are not required on a daily basis. Deficiencies are rare, while excesses of A and D can be toxic.

- Water-soluble vitamins, C and B complex, which include thiamin (B-1), riboflavin (B-2) niacin, pyridoxine (B-6), cyanocobalamin (B-12), folic acid, pantothenic acid, and biotin, are not stored in fat, and deficiencies can occur within two to four weeks. Excesses are eliminated in the urine, making toxicity rare.

- Certain vitamins such as C and E, and beta-carotene, which is metabolized as A, are potent antioxidants, protecting the cells against free radicals.

Vitamin C has often been referred to as the "Miracle Vitamin." Previously considered a great cold-fighter, it is now thought of as very advantageous to anti-aging. Jean Carper shares 15 ways that vitamin C may stop aging and extend life. Vitamin C:

- Suppresses high blood pressure
- Raises good–type HDL cholesterol
- Reduces bad-type LDL cholesterol as well as LP (another blood lipid hazard)
- Boosts levels of the body's most potent free radical enemy—glutathione
- Inhibits bad-type LDL cholesterol from becoming toxic (rancid or oxidized) and able to clog arteries
- Cleans fatty deposits from artery walls
- Strengthens blood vessel walls, preventing bruising
- Reduces the chance of heart attack–inducing vascular spasms
- Improves immune functioning
- Cuts odds of asthma, chronic bronchitis, and other lung and breathing problems

- Prevents periodontal disease by fending off free radical attacks on gum tissue
- Hinders oxidative damage to eyes, warding off cataracts and other age-related eye diseases
- Protects sperm from free radical damage causing birth defects
- Restores fertility in men
- Fights cancer by thwarting formation of carcinogens, blocking free radical DNA damage (which is a first step to cancer), preventing genes and viruses from switching on cancer activity, regulating immunity, and slowing tumor growth.

Minerals

- Minerals are inorganic elements essential to life.
- Minerals are involved in cellular and energy metabolism.
- Minerals act as enzymes or co-enzymes to regulate chemical reactions.
- Minerals are important for muscle contraction.
- Minerals are involved in the formation of teeth, bones, and hemoglobin, as well as in protein synthesis and hormone development.
- Major minerals, such as calcium, phosphorous, magnesium, potassium, sodium, and chloride have a daily requirement of more than 100 milligrams.
- Trace minerals are needed in quantities of less than 100 milligrams per day and are present in small quantities in the body.
- While theoretically it is possible to obtain all the required vitamins and minerals from a well-balanced diet, as a practical matter, unless you eat your fruits and vegeta-

bles straight from your garden, a great deal of the nutrition is lost in the packaging, storage, shipping, and cooling of foods.

Fiber

- Fiber forms the structural wall of plants.
- Fiber is technically not a nutrient since it is not digested.
- Fiber is found in fresh fruits and vegetables, whole grains, nuts, seeds, and legumes.
- Fiber bulks the stools and speeds the removal of waste products through the intestinal tract and out of the body.
- Fiber soaks up fat, fills the stomach, and cuts the appetite.
- Fiber reduces the risk of colon and other gut cancers.
- Water-soluble fiber comes mostly from whole-wheat products and increases the bulk in the digestive tract for faster elimination.
- Water-insoluble fiber, which includes beans and oat bran, has a high binding activity and is believed to lower serum cholesterol.
- The National Cancer Institute recommends 25 to 40 grams of fiber per day as opposed to the typical American intake of 18 to 20 grams per day. You need both water-soluble and water-insoluble fiber.

Water

- Water is the most essential nutrient for life.
- We can survive weeks without food, but only for a few days without water.
- Two-thirds of the body and 85 percent of the brain is water.
- Water is vital to almost every biological process,

including digestion, absorption, circulation, and excretion.

- Water is the main constituent of blood and lymph.
- Water regulates body temperature.
- Water lubricates joints and organs.
- Water moisturizes the skin.
- Water maintains strong muscle.
- Dehydration, especially in heat and during exercise, causes loss of electrolytes, such as potassium and sodium, and can be life threatening in advanced stages.
- We need a little over two quarts a day of water, or eight to ten eight-ounce glasses of water a day. Replenishing water is especially important after exercise.
- Drinking a glass of water before meals cuts the appetite.
- Drinking steam-distilled water has the added benefits of absorbing and eliminating toxins from the body.[1]

SOY

I can't discuss the elements of good nutrition without mentioning soy. Soy, a food product that's finding its way into many people's diets, is being dubbed, "a nutritional superstar." Soy has no cholesterol or saturated fat, but has plenty of protein, vitamins, and fiber. By studying soy-eating populations throughout the world, researchers have become aware of the vast health benefits derived from eating soy foods. These are some of the benefits attributable to soy according to Barry Sears, Ph.D., in his book *The Soy Zone*:

- Reduction of Heart Disease Risk: It's well known that in countries where soy products are eaten regularly, rates of heart disease are low.

- Protection Against Breast Cancer: Breast cancer occurs much less commonly in Asian countries where diets are rich in soy.

- Reduction of Prostate Cancer Risk: Rates of prostate cancer mortality are lower in Japanese males (who consume large amounts of soy/tofu) than in American males.

- Diminishing of Menopausal Symptoms: Recent research has shown that soy foods may be able to ease most menopausal symptoms, such as night sweats and hot flashes. In one study, night sweats and hot flashes were reduced by 40 percent in women who ate soy foods. Soy contains compounds (isoflavones) that can act as estrogen to help compensate for decreased natural estrogen production during menopause.

- Prevention of Osteoporosis: It has been shown that a diet rich in soy protein decreases the rate of bone loss. In one study, soy protein consumption actually increased bone density.

- Anti-Aging Benefits: One of the best things you can do to liven up your cells is to implant them with the substances found in soybeans. Some experts believe soybeans are the equivalent of an anti-aging pill. Dr. Denham Harman, the father of the free radical theory of aging, discovered a couple of decades ago that soybeans could interfere with free radical damage, which is at the heart of how fast you age.

Tofu, the king of traditional soy products, is protein-rich and extremely versatile. Also known as soybean curd, Tofu is a soft cheese-like food made by curdling fresh hot soymilk with a coagulant. Depending upon the amount of liquid extracted from the curds, the tofu is labeled as soft, medium, firm, or extra-firm. The firmer the tofu, the higher the protein to carbo-hydrate ratio.[2]

OTHER NUTRITIONAL HELPS

There are additional nutritional products on the market, which have proven valuable in achieving and maintaining a healthy lifestyle.

Noni Juice

Noni juice, which is used in a variety of products, has proven very beneficial to health improvement. Noni or (Nonu) is fruit of the Morinda Citrifolia plant, found mainly in the South Pacific (Tahiti) but it is also found in Indonesia, Taiwan, Philippines, Vietnam, India, Africa, Fiji, Guam, Hawaiian Islands and the West Indies. The plant was an important source of nourishment for ancient Polynesia. Every aspect of the plant was utilized as a food or medicinal source including the seeds, leaves, bark and roots.

It's physical characteristics are not exceedingly beautiful but as we know looks can be deceiving, for what Noni lacks in beauty it easily makes up for in nutritional and medicinal value.

A myriad of uses as cited by the International Noni Communication Council are attributed the xeronine molecule, (which some authorities say is the cell's best friend), which may be able along with its precursor of Proxeronine to become a protein source capable of multiple fundamental options and uses including the following:

• Parts of the fruit are used as a tonic and to control fever in China, Japan, and Hawaii.

• In the Pacific Islands, and Hawaii the leaves, flowers, fruit, and bark are used to treat eye problems, skin wounds and abscesses, gum and throat problems, respiratory ailments, constipation, and fever.

• In the Marshall Islands many use noni to treat stomach pains and after delivery.

• Juice of the leaves is taken for arthritis in the Philippines.

• In Indochina the fruit is taken for lumbago, asthma and dysentery.

• Pounded, unripe fruit mixed with salt is often applied to cuts and broken bones.

• Hawaiian's use the juices of over-ripe fruit to draw out pus from an infected boil.

• The fruit can also be used to make shampoo and to treat head lice.

A study by Mian-Ying Wang, M.D. shows that 86 percent of patients taking noni for various health problems experienced positive benefits.

Noni, an ancient mystery whose time has come—and perhaps is a new source to conquer many of life's maladies.

Aloe Vera

Aloe Vera, often referred to as *"The Potted Physician,"* has external as well as internal applications. Aloe, native to Africa, is also known as "lily of the desert," the "plant of immortality," and the "medicine plant." African hunters still rub the gel on their bodies to reduce perspiration and their scent.

Extensive research since the 1930s has shown that the clear gel has a dramatic ability to heal wounds, ulcers and burns by putting a protective coating on the affected areas and speeding up the healing rate. Aloe can also aid in keeping the skin supple, and has been used in the control of acne and eczema. It can help relieve itching due to insect bites and allergies. Aloe's healing power comes from increasing the availability of oxygen to the skin, and by increasing the synthesis and strength of tissue.

The plant is about 96 percent water. The rest of it contains active ingredients including essential oil, amino acids, minerals, vitamins, enzymes and glycoproteins. Many liquid health treatments are made from aloe, some combining aloe juice with other plants and herbs. The juice is soothing to digestive tract irritations, such as colitis and peptic ulcers.

As a food supplement, aloe is said to facilitate digestion, aid in blood and lymphatic circulation, as well as kidney, liver and gall bladder functions. Aloe contains at least three anti-inflammatory fatty acids that are helpful for the stomach, small intestine and colon. It naturally alkalizes digestive juices to prevent overacidity, a common cause of indigestion. It also helps cleanse the digestive tract by exerting a soothing, balancing effect.

A newly discovered compound in aloe, acemannan, is currently being studied for its ability to strengthen the body's natural resistance. Studies have shown acemannan to boost T-lymphocyte cells that aid the immune system.

Some are finding nutritional insurance for adults and children alike with the use of Protein drinks made with orange juice, or soy protein-based shakes. Nutritional supplements are a must to ensure your body has all the stress-fighting protection it needs. Help can be found in herbal tablets that provide a balance of essential vitamins and minerals while Vitamin C and bioflavonids support the adrenal glands

Ginseng
Siberian Ginseng supports the working of the adrenal glands and prevents the worst effects of nervous tension. It tends to increase energy, extend endurance and fight fatigue.

Siberian Ginseng also boosts overall immune function and may play a role in the treatment of hypertension, blood sugar irregularities and depression. Siberian Ginseng remedies are derived from the roots and sometimes from the leaves.

Studies on Siberian Ginseng have shown that it has considerable promise for increasing longevity and improving overall health. Chemists have isolated more than three dozen compounds in Siberian Ginseng that may affect the mind and body; foremost among these are the eleutherosides, which occur in the plant's roots and to a lesser degree, in the leaves.

Green Tea

One cup of herbal tea a day (preferably green tea) has been found in numerous studies to protect against cancer, especially lung cancer. Green tea is rich in polyphenol compounds known as catechins. These are not only responsible for the characteristic taste and color of tea, but are also thought to be responsible for many of the health benefits.

Catechins have antioxidant properties and may reduce body damage caused by free radicals. Higher consumption of green tea has been associated with a reduction in risk for heart disease and cancer, both of which may be related to free radical stress.

Bilberry Root

The anthocyanosides in bilberries can improve circulation, protect fragile capillaries and cause biochemical reactions in the eye; they have a positive effect on enzymes shown to alleviate symptoms of diabetes and heart disease. Although scientists don't know which components of the bilberry leaf are responsible for these effects, recent research has shown that taking a dried leaf extract will cause a drop in glucose (blood sugar) levels. The same research also showed that bilberry leaf can lower blood triglyceride levels, a heart disease risk factor.

Maca Root

Maca is a plant that grows in the mountains of Peru. It contains minerals, fatty acids and essential amino acid. These items are essential to proper cell, organ and transport systems of the body.

Guggul Extract

Guggul has a wide range of usefulness in indigenous medicine. It is an astringent and antiseptic. Guggul reduces cholesterol and triglycerides. It increases HDL cholesterol. It also resolves acne, reduces benign prostate enlargement, reduces inflammation of arthritis, is a thyroid stimulant, and helps improves heart disease by reducing platelet aggregation.

Yucca Root

Yucca root functions primarily for osteoarthritis and rheumatoid arthritis. Chemists and doctors speculate that the yucca saponins blocks the release of toxins from the intestinal tract which inhibits normal formation of cartilage. There may be anti-tumor factor as well yet studies on animals have been inconclusive.

Ginkgo Biloba

Ginkgo, stimulates brain activity by increasing levels of dopamine and improves the flow of blood to the brain and all other organs by dilating or relaxing the arteries and veins. Rich in flavonoids, antioxidants that protect the body against free radicals, ginkgo has also been shown to prevent blood clots by inhibiting blood cells from sticking together.

Pyruvate

Science has a way of surprising us with new and very interesting and appealing compounds to aid health. The latest and most effective is Pyruvate, a three carbon compound found in the body at all times. Once formed it goes to work immediately, acting at the level of the mitochondrion, or the "powerhouse" of the cell. Pyruvate is found in red apples, red wine, and certain cheeses. It may play a dramatic role in lowering the rate of heart disease. It is linked to the reduction of chronic diseases like cancer and heart disease. Research on the vast benefits of pyruvate is based on nearly three decades of research by Dr. Ronald Stanko, M.D. of the University of Pittsburgh. In his book *The Power of Pyruvate*, Dr. Stanko lists the following pluses of pyruvate:

1. Enhancement of fat loss and weight loss with weight reduction therapy
2. Prevention of fat gain and weight gain with overeating
3. Enhancement of exercise capacity
4. Inhibition of production of free radicals. Free radicals have been implicated as damaging agents in many diseases such as cancer, heart disease, and arthritis (See the "Four Basic Theories of Aging" on page 15)
5. Scavenging of free radicals
6. Inhibition of cancer growth
7. Inhibition of ischemic heart injury
8. Inhibition of ischemic intestinal injury
9. Decrease in heart damage after a heart attack
10. Decrease in blood cholesterol with consumption of a high-fat diet
11. Increase in heart muscle efficiency (the heart is able to pump blood without needing or using as much oxygen)
12. Decrease in the blood glucose in diabetes
13. Decrease in diabetic eye disease

14. Increase in cellular energy

15. Inhibition of cell death

16. Prevention of DNA damage

17. Inhibition of injury due to transplanted organs

18. Inhibition of injury to organs being readied for transplant while outside the body

With all these pluses, it is easy to see why pyruvate supplements are considered a great weapon in the armament against the disease of aging and in the pursuit of the forever factor.

When you consider that what we put in our mouths can make such a difference to the length and quality of the lives we live, it makes sense to develop a "carpe diem" mindset and to be willing to make good food choices, starting today. If you have been a "carpe cras" type of thinker in the past, always content to leave until tomorrow what you should be doing today, now is the time to change. As Benjamin Franklin wisely said, "A misty morning doesn't signify a cloudy day." In the past you may have made poor food choices, adversely affecting your health and shortening your life. However, today is a new day. Make the most of it!

WEIGHT LOSS

Being overweight or obese is a leading cause of preventable deaths in the United States today, being second only to smoking-related fatalities. These alarming facts are not too surprising when you realize research has shown that carrying excess weight will dramatically increase your risk of developing serious medical conditions, such as asthma, diabetes, hypertension, sleep apnea, arthritis, heart disease, cancer, and stroke.

In the fight against obesity, the first step is to assess your

BMI (Body Mass Index), which helps determine your potential risk for excess weight. While your primary care physician is an excellent resource for precise information, the following is a simple method for estimating your BMI:

Multiply your weight (in pounds) by 704.5.
Multiply your height (in inches) by your height (in inches).
Divide the first result by the second.

Example: If you're 5'5" and weigh 140 pounds:
140 x 704.5 = 98,630
65 x 65 = 4,225
98,630 divided by 4,225 = 23

Generally speaking, a score below 20 is very good, and potentially even underweight. A score between 20 and 25 is healthy, and a score above 25 is overweight.

Once you've determined what your BMI is, you can see if there is need for improvement. If you are overweight, *now* is the time to start doing something about it. In the words of David Hemmings: "If it isn't happening, make it happen." You need to eat a healthy diet, engage in a sensible exercise program, and utilize behavioral modifications, such as avoiding specific actions that trigger overeating.

If you are experiencing a weight problem, the first thing you need to do is alter your eating habits. A weight loss supplement may offer the needed assistance to achieve your goals. It is critical, however, that you are extremely careful when choosing a weight loss product. Many of them contain harmful ingredients such as ephedra and ma huang—stimulants which have led to a number of strokes and deaths. Fortunately, there are safe, sensible alternatives available.

The best weight loss products are the ones that address mood vs. food reaction, targeting emotional eaters. Such supplements attack weight problems by actually decreasing the desire to eat. One important thing to look for are ingredients such as pyridoxine, chromium picolonate that regulate insulin and stimulate serotonin levels. Serotonin is a chemical which gives us a sense of well-being and satisfaction. Other helpful ingredients are citrus aurantium, guarana, Pyruvate, vitamin B3, Vitamin B6, and gamma linolenic acid, which help decrease fat levels, increase feelings of satisfaction, enhance digestion, and regulate cholesterol levels.

If you are one of the millions of Americans who need to reduce caloric intake in order to promote weight loss, there are several very good weight loss programs available that emphasize healthy eating to lose weight. Recent research has shown that, rather than consuming the traditional three meals a day, eating several healthy small meals a day with a low glycemic index will reap the following benefits:

- Lowered stimulation of fat storage
- Reduction of appetite
- Enhanced sports performance
- Improved muscle to fat ratio
- Increased mental alertness
- Lowered caloric intake

Low glycemic food plans, which are based on high fiber, low fat, complex carbohydrate foods, also have been proven to reduce the incidence of type I diabetes and to help control type I and II diabetes, hypoglycemia, and hypertension. (Please visit **www.foreverfactor.com** for more information on glycemic index tests.)

A healthy diet and good nutrition are the foundation for an anti-aging lifestyle. Just as a car requires good fuel to run well, the human body functions according to the fuel it's given. Poor nutrition leads to poor performance; while a nutritious, varied diet promotes good health and a long life.

Forever Facts:

Remember: Approximately 127 million adults are overweight and the scale is rising in obesity in children. Obesity claims lives!

Change in eating habits is a key to maintaining a healthy lifestyle.

If you need to lose weight, cut calories slowly.

Avoid crash diets.

Take time to write down what you eat. It is surprising how many calories slip by in a day.

Eat plenty of fruits and vegetables.

Read labels and make low fat food choices.

Remember fiber keeps the body machinery running well and include plenty of fiber in your diet.

Antioxidants are key to anti-aging. Take vitamin and mineral supplements.

Don't skimp on water. Stay thirsty and healthy.

Weight problems claimed 350,000 lives in the United States last year alone.

Endnotes:

1. Nutritional information on Carbohydrates, Fats, Proteins, Vitamins, Minerals, Fiber, and Water derived from Dr. Ronald Klatz's book *Grow Young with HGH*.

2. Soy information derived from the book *The Soy Zone* by Barry Sears, Ph.D.

"You've reached middle age when all you
exercise is caution."
—Unknown

Exercising Your Options

Spencer W. Kimball, a great religious leader, kept a small plaque on his desk that portrayed the two-word motto he lived by: "Do It!" He urged his followers to also "Do It," encouraging them to prioritize, set goals, and then follow through; to not be content with simply discussing goals or planning goals, but to actually do what needed to be done. Later, a sports company added the word "Just" to the "Do It" idea, and its slogan of "Just Do It" is recognized world-wide.

The "Just Do It" ideology is in sync with anti-aging philosophy, particularly as it applies to exercise programs and getting into shape physically. Consider this all too familiar scenario:

A man is in terrible physical condition. He's overweight and out of shape. Determined to do something about it, he goes to the mall to look at exercise equipment. A clerk asks if she can assist him, and the man says he want to buy a stair climber. He is told that all exercise equipment is on the second floor. He declines the stairs and asks for the elevator with the comment, "I don't feel like walking up to see it."

This mind-set and wishy-washy commitment to physical improvement is responsible for many of the aches and pains of aging. Being sedentary is a problem of aging, and exercise is the well-documented solution.

In his article, "Promoting and Prescribing Exercise for the Elderly" in the February 2002 issue of *American Family Physician*, Robert J. Nied summarizes some of the health gains attributable to exercise. The best known advantages of exercise are cardiovascular benefits, which include improved blood pressure, lipid profiles (*lipids are various substances, such as fats, that, along with proteins and carbohydrates, make up the principal structural parts of living cells*), and functioning of the cardiorespiratory system. Exercise-related improvements are also tied to type 2 diabetes, which include generally lowered incidence, improved sensitivity to insulin, and improved sugar control. Osteoporosis studies of exercise show reduced bone loss in postmenopausal women, a decrease in hip and vertebral fractures, and a lowered risk of falling. Arthritis-related improvements from exercise include improved function and decreased pain. Improvements are also noted in neurologic/emotional health, namely improved sleep quality, better cognitive function, less depression, and better short-term memory function. In summary, Nied ties exercise to a decreased risk of obesity and to a general reduction in rates of illness and death.

As illustrated above, exercise, in its various forms, can have dramatic benefits in numerous areas of life, health, and function, due to its impact on various body systems. Exercise should not be viewed as a panacea, however, nor should it be viewed as "medicine" without potential side effects. Physical Therapist Trent Casper reminds, "Exercise, to be effective and successful, must be appropriate to your prescribed needs. **As with medication, it is recommended to consult with one's personal physician before beginning any exercise program, where an exercise prescription can be discussed.**"

A good friend of mine, Alison Taglianetti, fitness expert,

shares the following information about an individualized exercise program/prescription. Allison says such a program should include the following components:

- Aerobic/anaerobic conditioning,
- Muscular strength and endurance
- Flexibility and relaxation.

To further promote the effectiveness of the individualized exercise program, each of the above components should include the parameters of **frequency (F)** of the activity, **intensity (I)** of the activity, **time (T)** or duration of the activity and **type (T)** or mode of the activity in the planning phase of a fitness program. All together, these four parameters are appropriately referred to as **FITT** and are detailed below. Beyond the FITT factors, special consideration should also be given to the following characteristics of the participant:

- Present fitness level
- Orthopedic limitations
- Obesity or other weight related limitations
- Cardiovascular disease, arthritis, etc.
- Accessibility to fitness centers, equipment, walking trails, etc.

CARDIOVASCULAR CONDITIONING

Cardiovascular (CV) conditioning can be sub-categorized into aerobic and anaerobic conditioning. Aerobic exercise refers to activity performed in the presence of oxygen, utilizing fat stores as the main source of energy. Aerobic endurance or conditioning provides the foundation for all future fitness achievement and, thereby, is the primary focus of a successful exercise program. Again, specifying the FITT parameters for aerobic conditioning is greatly influenced by the present fitness level or status of the individual. For those that are new to exercise, starting off cautiously and comfortably is crucial in the long-term physical effectiveness of the activity. In regard to Frequency of aerobic CV conditioning, the general recommendation is to participate in activities five to seven times per week. For the true novice to exercise, perhaps this guideline begins with three CV sessions per week with the goal of progressively adding extra sessions as one is mentally and physically ready. It should be stressed that, independent of one's fitness level, starting an exercise program on the moderate side (both mentally and physically) is highly recommended. All too often we start overzealously with exercise only to get injured, burnt-out, and/or so frustrated with the time-constraints of this new activity that we abruptly quit. Easing into exercise is the best advice.

Intensity of the CV aspect of one's program is perhaps of utmost importance. Aerobic conditioning guidelines recommend that this activity fall into the intensity of 60–85 percent of one's maximal heart rate (HR). What does this mean? The ideal method of determining one's maximal heart rate is under the supervision of a cardiologist during a Cardiovascular Stress Test. While we are not all required to have this test done, there are other means by which we can establish personalized heart rate zones (target HR zones) for aerobic conditioning. The simplest method is utilizing the following formula:

220–age = Estimated Max HR

Estimated Max HR x 60 percent = Lower End of Personalized Training/Target HR Zone (A)

Estimated Max HR x 85 percent = Upper End of Personalized Training/Target HR Zone (B)

Zone "A" to "B" = HR zone within which one should exercise to achieve aerobic benefit.

The "A" to "B" zone is more specifically the range of estimated heartbeats per minute to achieve aerobic/CV benefit. Monitoring one's HR can be done easily by counting the number of beats/pulses one feels in a one minute time frame on the upper left hand side of the back of the wrist (below the thumb) and comparing this number to the above range. For true effectiveness, the purchase of a HR monitor is highly recommended. These easy-to-use devices can be found in any sporting goods store and can provide a wealth of information and motivation to the participant.

There are many problems with the above formula in the sense that it only considers the age factor of the participant. There are no considerations given to fitness level, cardiovascular impairments, obesity, orthopedic limitations, prescription medications, etc. So how do we take the above simple formula and personalize it to one's true intensity recommendation?

The answer lies in the addition of a Perceived Exertion Scale (PES) to this formula. The PES is the exercise participant's personal classification or "tuning in" as to how hard they feel the exercise intensity actually is—how hard they perceive their exertion to be. Again for simplicity, we recommend a PES of 1-10 with "1" being extremely easy (i.e. lying on the couch wiggling your big toes) while "10" is extremely exhausting (i.e. any activity that causes excessive winding and is difficult to maintain for more than 30-60 seconds).

An effective PES for aerobic conditioning would have the participant on a scale of "5" to "8." Cross-referencing one's Target HR zone with the PES will provide an individualized "A" to "B" zone as a guideline for aerobic conditioning. There is no greater tool in the ultimate success to any exercise program than the ability of "tuning in" on how you feel during exercise. If something feels too heavy, too hard, too fast, too long, or whatever measure you are considering when you exercise, it is better to err on the side of caution. Remember to perform the talk test. While exercising, you should be able to talk when you need to, but you shouldn't be able to carry on a nonstop conversation. Your heart rate and need for oxygen should be elevated, but you shouldn't be gasping for air. Let me reiterate, tune in to how you feel!

Time, or duration, of the aerobic component is between 20 to 60 minutes per session. As a reminder, the recommendation for Frequency of CV conditioning is ultimately 5 to 7 sessions per week. The goal of aerobic conditioning is to increase the time per session and number of sessions per week while maintaining a PES rating of 5 to 8 for the entire activity. Again, there are always considerations. If excess weight is a health concern, we unquestionably want to work on increasing the amount of time per session with less emphasis on the higher end of the PES. If time constraints are a concern, then we need to limit the minutes per session but perhaps work on increasing the PES to a 7 or 8 to compensate.

Type or mode of the aerobic aspect of one's program refers to the selection of walking, jogging, running, stair-climbing, bicycling, etc. It is SO important to choose an activity that you enjoy! Remember, the benefits of exercise come through consistency as well as effectiveness. No one wants to do something they don't enjoy or something that hurts or bothers them physically. Ideally, changing the mode of training, more commonly referred to as cross-training, has tremendous benefits. For example, combining a walking program with a stair-climbing routine uses the musculature differently, providing additional benefits; or, choosing a flat walking route one day and switching to a hilly route the next will net additional advantages.

Another key to a successful exercise program is to add diversity. Diversity can be applied across the entire FITT recommendations by taking a longer, less intense walk (60-minutes, PES=5) one day and then a shorter, more intense walk the next (30-minutes, PES=8). The body adapts very quickly. Spice up your exercise regimen and reap greater rewards.

Anaerobic conditioning is any activity conducted at a target HR zone of 85 percent to approximately 92 percent of one's estimated Max HR. On the PES scale, this activity would be a "9" or "10." Considering the intensity of the activity, this is not a recommended component for those exercisers who are classified as beginner to intermediate. For those above the intermediate level of fitness, incorporating one to two sessions of anaerobic training into a weekly program will ultimately enhance one's overall cardiovascular conditioning. Due to the intensity of this component, the time factor rapidly declines to an activity that one can maintain for less than a two-minute period. Type, or mode, follows the same guidelines as in the aerobic category.

MUSCULAR STRENGTH AND ENDURANCE

The inclusion of a muscular strength and endurance component to an exercise program has a number of benefits. The true goal of any exercise program is to enhance the quality of one's life by providing the endurance and stamina to participate in the daily activities/tasks of one's life with ease. A well-rounded muscular strength and endurance (MSE) program will provide the strength to perform daily chores and hobbies, enhance metabolism thru increased muscle mass, assist in the prevention of orthopedic injury, assist in the maintenance of joint health or integrity and enhance the cosmetic appearance of muscle tone in the participant.

The basic guidelines for implementing an effective MSE program are the following:

- Include exercises that target the chest, shoulders, upper and lower back, abdominal area, hips, buttocks, quadriceps, hamstrings, and calf muscles.

- Per session, choose one exercise per target area (as listed above) and perform 1-2 sets of 15+/-repetitions per set.

- Select a weight/resistance that can be performed thru a full range of movement (complete extension to complete flexion) in a slow-controlled motion to a comfortable point of fatigue at the completion of the set.

- As a recommendation, apply a slow 4-count in each direction of the exercise (extension and flexion) and add a brief end point at the full extension point and the full flexion point of the exercise.

- Increase the weight/resistance only as the sensation of "comfortable fatigue" begins to diminish, providing the timing and range of motion factors are preserved.

- As mentioned in the CV component, add diversity thru incorporating different exercises that target the same muscle. For example, choose a rowing exercise for the upper back one day and then a lateral pull down exercise for your next MSE session that week.

This MSE component can be added safely and effectively to one's program by applying, again, the factors of FITT. In the Frequency arena, the recommendation is for MSE activities to be performed 2-3 times per week, including exercises that target the back, chest, shoulders, abdominal, hips/buttocks, quadriceps, hamstrings, and calf muscles during each session. It is beneficial to try to evenly space these MSE sessions throughout the week, if possible. The Frequency component takes on a secondary meaning in the MSE category in respect to the timing of the movement and the number of repetitions performed for each exercise. A repetition refers to the number of times a specific exercise is performed without rest. General recommendations for the repetition factor, or frequency parameter, would be to perform two sets per major muscle group with 15 repetitions per set as mentioned above.

The Intensity factor includes selecting a weight or resistance that can be performed thru a full range of motion to a comfortable point of fatigue. Lifting a weight or resistance that is too heavy will cause the range of motion to be hindered which will have negative effects on using MSE exercises to promote joint strength and flexibility.

Time, in the component of MSE, would refer to the overall plan of incorporating weight/resistance programming into one's routine 2-3 times per week. This factor would also include the timing guidelines of each repetition. As previously stated, each repetition should be performed in a slow-controlled movement with a recommendation of a four count in each direction of flexion and extension. Time can be included again in consideration of taking an approximately 30-second rest between muscle sets.

Lastly, Type or mode is best pulled into our program design by the decision or availability of actual strength training machines, free weights, resistance tubing or bands, or calisthenics exercises. Ideally, access to strength training equipment and an exercise specialist or certified personal trainer enhances the effectiveness of this component. Resistance bands, however, are affordable and convenient. Whatever the mode, emphasis again is placed on diversity and changing up exercises per muscle group. Changing between weight equipment, resistance bands, calisthenics, etc. would be ideal at spicing the program up, making it a bit more fun and creative and adding the "change" that one's body needs to improve.

FLEXIBILITY AND RELAXATION

One of the key factors to enhancing the quality of life through exercise is maintaining joint integrity and flexibility. In order for a muscle to move effectively, it needs to be pliable and elastic—not rigid and tight. Incorporating a flexibility aspect into one's program allows for greater ease in movement and reduces the potential for injury. Physical injuries can occur both muscularly as well as from an orthopedic standpoint. Therefore, a program that comfortably stretches all the major muscle groups of the body in their entirety is highly recommended. Once again, lets apply the FITT principles.

Frequency in flexibility is unquestionably mandatory. As with aerobic conditioning, a complete flexibility routine should be performed 5 to 7 days per week. The program should work at elongating all the major muscles of the upper and lower back, chest, shoulders, abdomen, hips and buttocks, quadriceps, hamstrings and lower leg muscles. Participants should perform one stretching exercise per muscle group, repeating each stretch two times. All stretching exercises should be held in the position where the participant reaches a comfortable point of pull for a slow, steady count of ten.

Intensity of stretching, as just stated, should always be within a comfort zone. Stretching has a number of physical as well as emotional benefits. Approaching each flexibility exercise with this mind set will provide a more effective outcome to this component of one's program. Stretching should never be done to a point of pain or discomfort. The participant should always be able to rhythmically breathe throughout the entire 10-count stretch. Repeating each stretch will allow the participant to "sink" a little deeper into the stretch and thereby enhance the elongation aspect of this component.

The Time considerations of a flexibility program are minimal. A complete stretching program can be conducted in under 20-minutes, providing the 10-count per exercise and the two time repetition is applied. Depending on the participant's goals, incorporating a yoga or stretch class that is more focused on the flexibility aspect might be advisable. These classes generally last an hour and are quite comprehensive in overall flexibility.

The Type parameter opens many doors. Thankfully, the trend in the fitness industry has moved us toward activities that include more flexibility and relaxation principles. It is extremely easy to get involved in a yoga, Pilates, or Tai Chi class. Again, the encouragement is toward diversity and implementing as many different techniques as possible.

The proper implementation of the exercise parameters discussed above will influence the success of your exercise program.[1]

In an article in the *Journal of Anti-Aging Medicine*, Dr. Robert Goldman reminds us that "exercise is often referred to as the ultimate anti-aging pill." He is an advocate of everyone at every age engaging in some form of physical activity. Dr. Goldman suggests that exercise does not just help the body physically, but also mentally, emotionally, and socially.

I agree with experts who feel exercise is a valuable weapon in the anti-aging arsenal. People who are physically fit, eat a healthy, balanced diet, and take nutritional supplements can measure out to be 10 to 20 years younger biologically than their chronological age, making them an immortal. Being an immortal in this sense doesn't mean living forever, but, instead, is defined as being free from mental and physical disease and degeneration for years longer than an unhealthy individual. Exercise is an extremely important part of achieving this immortality.

Remember, it doesn't matter if you were once physically active in your younger years. If you're not currently engaged in a physical activity program on a regular basis, your body is not receiving the innumerable health-related benefits available from exercise. Dr. Goldman reiterates the following reasons to exercise.

Exercise:
- Increases the body's ability to lose weight—especially fat weight
- Improves immune system functioning
- Betters body posture
- Reduces the risk of heart disease
- Improves the body's ability to use fat for energy during physical activity
- Aids the body in resisting upper-respiratory tract infections
- Relieves the pain of tension headaches
- Increases maximal oxygen intake
- Preserves lean body mass
- Improves coronary heart circulation
- Increases levels of HDL cholesterol and reduces LDL cholesterol
- Improves short-term memory
- Enhances sexual desire, performance, and satisfaction
- Improves quality of sleep
- Improves physical appearance
- Enhances self-esteem

- Generates more energy and vigor to meet the demands of daily life
- Increases overall health awareness
- Improves general mood

Remember with every exercise program, two important parts of your exercise session are the warm-up and the cool-down. Don't forget to stretch and warmup before doing any exercise. Warm up can be 5 minutes on a treadmill, pedaling on your bike at an easy pace, swimming a few slow laps, or jogging in place. The warm-up helps the blood flow to the muscles, which help them to relax and contract more smoothly. When you break a light sweat, it is time to begin. Afterward, remember to always cool down. It is a good idea to replenish lost fluid and nutrients by drinking one to two glasses of water after you exercise to replace lost fluids.

Outside of your formal exercise program, be alert for opportunities to add activity to your day. Park your car at the far end of the parking lot when you do your grocery shopping instead of near the door. Walk past the elevator and take the stairs. On your break at work, pass up the vending machine and go outside for a breath of fresh air and walk for 10 minutes. Give your body a break from sitting and blow the cobwebs away. You'll be more alert and ready to function after you come back inside. In recent years, scientists have determined that exercise adds up the way that calories do. Three 10-minute walks a day is considered as beneficial as one 30-minute walk.

There is no question as to the value of exercise in our lives. With all the advantages of exercise, it should definitely have a scheduled time on our daily calendars. So, if you're all psyched up and ready to start exercising, let me leave you with two final thoughts. George Elliott said, "It is never too late to become what you might have been." And finally, "Just Do It!"

Forever Facts:

Exercise reduces the risk of stroke.

There is an exercise to fit the needs and likes of everyone.

Exercise helps in the management of stress.

Exercise improves the quality of sleep.

It is never too late to start.

Inactivity speeds up the aging process.

Exercise doesn't have to be expensive to be effective.

Exercise reduces the risk of developing colon, breast, and prostrate cancer.

Consistency is the key with exercise.

Exercise helps alleviate depression.

Exercise relieves back pain and constipation.

Exercise protects against "creeping obesity," slow weight gain that occurs with age.

Exercise can stimulate libido.

You haven't failed at exercise until you have quit trying.

The typical American adult watches four hours of television everyday. If a mere thirty minutes of this time were devoted to moderate exercise (which could be done in front of the TV) the resulting health benefits would be tremendous.

Exercise programs offer a host of benefits to arthritis and fibromyalgia sufferers. It has been found to reduce joint pain and stiffness, build strong muscles around the joints, and increase flexibility and endurance.

Endnotes:

1. All "FITT" exercise information derived from Alison Casey Taglianetti, B.S., NSCA-CPT.

"The sexes were made for each other, and only in the wise and loving union of the two is the fullness of health and duty and happiness to be expected."
—Havelock Ellis

Wise and Loving Union

"There is nothing more important than SEX because without it, there is no life at all."
—Dr. Richard Schulze

About the time we reach 40, our bodies undergo profound changes that affect every aspect of our lives, including how we look, feel, think and, age. For most people, the first sign of aging is excessive fatigue. You often hear comments of "the old gray mare ain't what she used to be," or "I think I am running out of steam." This feeling is a likely description of exactly what is happening to our bodies, as the aging process takes place. The metabolism slows down, making it harder to burn calories, which results in stored fat, weight gain, and lost muscle tone.

Every activity—even breathing and thinking—requires energy. The energy shortage in mid-life affects every cell and system in our body. The heart, brain, and kidneys slow down. Cells lose their ability to repair themselves and die. Our immune system functions less efficiently, our endocrine system stops producing hormones at youthful levels, and our skin becomes drier. It is not surprising, then, that sexual functioning is likewise affected by the aging process.

Impotence is one of the problems that is oftentimes age related. There are many physical causes for temporary or chronic impotence, which can range from the easily avoidable or curable, to very severe causes, which cannot be cured without radical, invasive measures, such as surgery. Several years ago, it was thought that psychological factors were the primary cause of male impotence. Sex experts now believe that physical causes are responsible for about 75 percent of the cases of men over 50, caused by the same buildup of cholesterol plaques that narrow the coronary arteries and cause heart attacks.

According to an article in *Postgraduate Medicine* by J.E. Motley, male sexual dysfunction has been shown to be a preceding sign of heart attack or stroke. The same risk factors that contribute to heart disease, namely poor lipid profile, high cholesterol, low HDL and high LDL, high triglycerides, and cigarette smoking can contribute to impotence.

The following are some of the more common physical causes of impotence:

- Problems with the blood supply
- Side effect of medicines and drugs
- Disorders of the nervous system
- Hormonal disorders
- Other complex or multisystemic diseases

Women's hormone changes are far more sudden and dramatic than those experienced by men. As a whole, they have fewer sexual problems, and the problems they do have tend to be more easily remedied.

Menopause is caused by a decline in two key hormones: estrogen and progesterone. These are produced in women by the ovaries and the adrenal glands. After age thirty, the production of these hormones begins to slowly decline. Women in their 40's and 50's show a dramatic decline as the ovaries cease functioning and no longer produce estrogen. Progesterone production implicitly shuts down. Some women will feel no change, while others will experience unpleasant symptoms, including hot flashes, headaches, fatigue, insomnia, depression, as well as the loss of libido. The decline in estrogen and progesterone can leave women vulnerable to heart disease, osteoporosis, memory loss, thinning hair and other health problems. In checking with your physician, you will find there are many things available to help with these changes in both men and women. The important thing to remember is aging is *not* a lost cause.

There has never been a time in history when there is so much discussion about sex. Fulton J. Sheen observes: "Sex has become one of the most discussed subjects of modern times. The Victorians pretended it did not exist; the moderns pretend that nothing else [does]."

Everyone was more than mildly surprised when Bob Dole appeared in prime time TV commercials, touting products to help with erectile dysfunction. Figures and studies today show, however, that there are more men who are experiencing erectile dysfunction (ED) than ever before. Some doctors are finding the need for specialization in that field of medicine and are having much success. There are topical transactive serums designed specifically for treatment of impotence and erectile dysfunction. A nitric oxide activator helps in increasing blood flow and muscle tone. Ingredients which aid are:

- **Arginine**—an essential amino acid, which the body cannot manufacture from other substances.
- **Nitric Oxide**—which acts as an essential chemical trigger producing erections.
- **Gingko Biloba**—which works by increasing blood flow

and circulation, enhancing the nitric oxide levels, working synergistically with arginine.

- **Pyruvate**—may be one of the best sources to directly increase nitric oxide levels, which chemically induces erections.

There are other issues regarding sex and sexual behavior that are important to discuss. First, let's look at what Wendy and Larry Maltz call the Healthy Sex CERTS model. Healthy sex requires that these five basic conditions be met: Consent, Equality, Respect, Trust, and Safety.

Consent means you can freely and comfortably choose whether or not to engage in sexual activity. You are able to stop the activity at any time during the sexual contact.

Equality means your sense of personal power is on an equal level with your partner. Neither of you dominates the other.

Respect means you have positive regard for yourself and for your partner. You feel respected by your partner.

Trust means you trust your partner on both a physical and emotional level. You have mutual acceptance of vulnerability and an ability to respond to it with sensitivity.

Safety means you feel secure and safe within the sexual setting. You are comfortable with and assertive about where, when, and how the sexual activity takes place.

It takes spending time together and engaging in lots of honest, open communication to make sure that the CERTS conditions are operating in your relationship. That's just one reason why a strong friendship and commitment should precede sexual involvement.

One aid to assist an on-going sexual relationship is one

important to both men and women. In our busy lives we overlook and oftentimes forget the beauty of showing affection. An unexpected hug, a show of appreciation, and even a simple thank you does wonders to arouse the spirit.

In regard to having a healthy sex life, perhaps the most important thing we should remember is sex is not meant to be entertainment alone, but should be a result of affection and love. A tobacco advertisement suggests, "You've come a long way, baby." But is the long way a good way? Or, should we go back to the ways of those who set their goals to marry because of love and trust, seeing the sexual act as an expression of love, closeness and happiness—not just satisfaction of the moment?

Forever Facts:

Lack of exercise can reduce the sex drive. Great revivers are swimming, running, and bicycle riding.

We are never too old to show affection.

Kindness says, "I care and want to be close."

*"A weak mind is like a microscope, which magnifies trifling
things but cannot conceive great ones."*
—*Lord Chesterfield*

The Brain: Use It or Lose It

A sixty-five year old woman had an age scan performed,
where her cognitive functioning was tested. She tested very
poorly. Her doctor made several recommendations to her for
improvement. She decided to utilize his "use it or lose it"
suggestions for stimulating mental activity. This woman went
home and began memorizing. She memorized scriptural
passages, poems, sayings, etc. She practiced repeating to
herself anything she might want to remember, stimulating her
brain function. After sticking with her memorization program
for a number of months, she went back in for testing. Her
cognitive functioning was dramatically improved.

In their book *The Longevity Strategy*, David Mahoney and
Richard Restak point out:

> Every talent and special skill that you've developed
> over your lifetime is represented in your brain by a
> complex network of neurons . . . each time you engage
> in any activity that involves your talents and skills, the
> neuronal linkages in that network are enhanced. Think
> of the brain cells as shaped like trees composed of long
> branches subdividing into smaller and smaller
> branches. As a result of brain growth and the person's
> experience in the world, tremendous overlap and
> connectivity develop among the tree branches.

Eventually nerve cells form active circuits based on these branchlike linkages. The more often the circuits are activated, the easier it is to activate them the next time.

If you neglect your talents and skills that involve cognitive functioning, they begin to wane. Over time, it becomes harder and harder to perform at your best. I am convinced that the longer your brain is neglected, the harder it becomes to return to your same level of excellence. The reason for this is the neuronal circuits have fallen into disuse, requiring greater degrees of effort to activate them. There is one important thing to remember, however. No matter how long you neglect a skill or talent, it will still be easier for you to reclaim it than for one who has never learned such a skill or talent in the first place.

The brain is an ever-changing organ. If one part gets rusty and suffers atrophy from disuse, its functions are taken over by other areas that are used more. Some scientists believe that by using what you don't want to lose for only half an hour two to three times a week, you won't get rusty and will be able to maintain your skills and talents.

The following suggests we must be aware of so called brain drainers—complications to the brain that we bring on ourselves by our lifestyles.

Brain Drainers, a term used by Paul Yanick, Jr. and Vincent C. Giampapa in their book *Quantum Longevity* is consistent with lifestyle choices that have a negative impact on health and therefore on thinking, memory, and concentration. These brain drainers must be corrected or avoided in order for memory to function properly.

Smoking: Although low doses of nicotine can be a potent memory enhancer, the overall effect of smoking is clearly detrimental because of its effects on the lungs. Not only does smoking double your chances of suffering a heart attack, it constricts blood vessels, interfering with circulation throughout the body. When you smoke, the brain's oxygen supply is reduced, resulting in diminished mental function. Remember, once a brain cell is damaged it cannot be regenerated.

Alcohol: Of all the brain drainers, this is the worst. Drinking large quantities—more than two drinks a day—can inflict drastic damage to every organ of the body, including the brain. Alcohol depresses brain function, can alter personality, and can reduce a person's ability to concentrate, learn, and remember.

Obesity: Excessive weight and body fat can led to reduced overall mental functioning. Carrying too much weight puts a great burden on the circulatory system, inhibiting the most effective employment of blood sugars, which are crucial for maximal brain functioning. Obesity also causes sleep apnea, a potentially life-threatening disorder that constantly disrupts sleep. Cognition is adversely affected because a person with this condition has difficulty staying awake during the day, let alone thinking clearly.

Modern research suggests that we need to exercise our brain to stay healthy, youthful and strong. We know that such training has a profound impact on how much and how fast our brain ages—or, better, on how young it stays. The process of "cognitive training" is the best way to maximize our biological potential and keep our brains stronger and sharper longer.

The most exciting studies show that you can even reverse the brain's physical deterioration that may have already started! An extensive study by Stuart Berger M.D. includes a score of research papers that show continual brain training and learning can offset and even reverse brain aging. Older animals that live in rich and varied environments, with the opportunity for constant learning, actually show organic changes in their brains. The nerve connections grow more complex with more synapses and more closely resemble the brains of healthy younger animals.

Another study of four thousand older volunteers proves that many of them could greatly improve two kinds of brain skills that had declined with age, simply by using braining techniques. Two out of five subjects made so much progress that they actually regained the performance levels they had shown fourteen years earlier, in effect turning back the clock a decade and a half in their brain's functional age!

A report from a National Institute on Aging task force confirms that one in five older people with intellectual impairment may be able to reverse the downward slide.

Cognitive training was found to increase older people's accuracy on standard mental-function tests, so they scored as though they were "younger."

With these encouraging findings from research, we need to discover how to take advantage of this information and apply it to our own brains.

One good way is by taking tests designed to sharpen specific skills of spatial orientation and inductive reasoning. Research suggests that practicing on these tests can help you sharpen those skills and effectively lower the functional age of your brain. Just doing these tests one time won't, of course, take years off the age of your brain. It has been said, "You are what you repeatedly do." As with any learning process, the key is consistency. You need to build into your life these kind of challenging mental exercises on a regular basis.

Get in the habit of doing games, tests, quizzes, puzzles, or brain twisters. You can pick up a collection at your local bookstore. Scrabble, word jumbles, acrostics, and even crossword puzzles can give the brain necessary exercise. Card games are particularly helpful for training reasoning and retention.

Take a course at a local college or adult-education center. The practice you get in memorization, inductive or deductive reasoning, spatial orientation, or calculation will help give you the mental exercise you need.

Pick up any one of the scores of preparation books for the SAT or other standardized scholastic tests. They are treasure troves of exactly the kind of varied, stimulating mental exercises that can help your brain stay young.

If there is a university near you, its psychology department may have a specialist in psychometric testing. He or she may be able to help you obtain hundreds of brain-expanding tests and test instruments. Or, look in the "psychometrics" section of your local library for test instruments you can use as brain-training tools.

Be consistent in practicing whatever skill you choose. Work at the same time each day so the brain will be primed and ready to get the maximum out of each session.

Keep challenging yourself. Throw away your calculator. Remember those days in elementary school when the teachers would challenge you to add up columns of figures. Do that exercise again and again, along with others that cause you to use your mind and thought processes.

Learn something new. Have you ever wanted to learn French, master the computer, or write a short story? There's no time like the present to learn something new. Community colleges are great resources for classes to help stimulate the brain and bring about a feeling of rejuvenation.

I don't have to tell you that to keep any muscle strong and limber, you have to exercise it. The brain is no different. Use it. I endorse the following thought of Benjamin Franklin, and apply it to the brain. He said:

"You can't lose [it] until you quit trying."

<u>Forever Facts:</u>

Memorization is a very helpful brain training tool.

Never be afraid to learn something new.

Consistency and repetition are key elements in stimulating the brain.

Public libraries are treasure troves of brain-training materials.

Brain exercises have to challenge to be effective.

Dr. Stephen Lamm, M.D., in his book *Younger at Last*, lists certain medications or over-the-counter drugs that can affect mental sharpness and trigger short-term memory loss. They include:

- **Weight loss medications (e.g. Pondimin and Redux)**

- **Hypertension drugs (e.g. Aldomet and Inderal)**

- **Anti-depression drugs (e.g. Asendin, Elavil and Pamelor)**

- **Anti-anxiety medications (e.g. Dalmane, Serax and Valium)**

- **Anti-psychosis medications (e.g. Haldol, Mellaril and Thorazine)**

- **Diabetes (e.g. Insulin)**

- **Antacid medications (e.g. Pepcid, Tagamet and Zantac)**

- **Parkinson's disease medications (e.g. Symmetrel)**

"Intellectual blemishes, like facial ones, grow more prominent with age."
—Francois de la Rouchefoucauld

Putting Your Best Face Forward

Chances are if you tune into the news, via television, radio, internet, or newspaper on any given day, you will find at least one story, commercial, or advertisement related to aging. There might be stories on arthritis, heart disease, cancer, or other degenerative diseases and disorders associated with the aging process, highlighting the grim statistics attesting to our awful mortality. There might be commercials with companies touting their incontinence products for the elderly or ads for adult day care. Such media presentations are peppered with words and phrases associated with aging such as: taking pills, dyeing hair, fading memory, false teeth, bifocal lenses, grumpy, hard of hearing, retiring, thinning hair, wrinkles, and osteoporosis. Is it any wonder that getting older doesn't seem a pleasant prospect to anyone?

Thinking about aging, a little boy kept observing his grandmother and finally asked her if her wrinkles hurt. She patiently started to explain, "Oh no, this is just what happens to us when we grow up and start to get old." Before she could finish explaining, her grandson quickly interrupted, "Well, if that's what you get for growing up, I guess I'll just stay a kid."

Obviously, no one wants the apparent signs of aging or the health complications that usually accompany the aging process. These feelings, however, are not new.

We can go back in history to the 16th century and spot a

Spanish galleon appearing off the coast of the Florida penin-
sula. On the decks, the famed Spanish explorer Ponce de Leon
senses that he is within days of completing his sacred mission.
As the ship rolls gently beneath his feet, he scans the horizon.
He has heard tell that on these shores exists a secret fount.
Revered by the Indians in the region, its waters are rumored to
have mysterious properties conferring lasting vigor, beauty,
and youth to all who drink them. His quest, de Leon knows, is
to claim the fountain for Spain's King, Ferdinand II, and to
bring that elixir home to the royal families of Europe.

Just as Ponce de Leon searched for the fountain of youth,
we are in search of the "forever factor." While the dream of
never aging is not realistic, I know that adding years to life and
life to years is a viable reality. There are scientists today in their
laboratories who are finding just what Ponce de Leon only
dreamed of. Albert Rosenfeld wrote in *Prolongevity*:

> Aging, as we have always known it, may no longer
> be inevitable or irrevocable. Breakthroughs all across
> the frontier of biomedical science make it increasingly
> feasible to hope that we may hold back the ravages of
> senescence—even to abolish many of the degenerative
> symptoms of the hitherto universal disease called old
> age. For nearly every symptom of aging...there are
> remedies and preventive measures being actively inves-
> tigated.

With this injection of hope into the prospect of aging, it is
time to forget the idea that aging must be destructive. I recommend we focus on ways to improve the aging process, helping
ourselves to look and feel better.

Whether we like it or not, much of our self-worth and
personal empowerment are ultimately related to how youthful

and vital we look. Appearance is the face we present to the world and, as such, is very important. Outward appearance is not just empty vanity, it is our passport to the world. It tells people who see us for the first time how we feel about ourselves.

The January 1988 editorial in the *Journal of the American Medical Association* states: "It is increasingly apparent that appearance, certainly including cutaneous [that relating to the skin] appearance, contributes to society's evaluation of an individual's competence and to that individual's sense of self worth and well-being....The prospect of [an] effective anti-aging product for the skin may have direct medical benefits beyond its effect on premalignant lesions." Or, to put it in layman's terms, experts realize that looking as young as you feel is a necessary part of being a vigorous, healthy person.

As a plastic surgeon, I can certainly verify the feelings a person experiences when they are able to see their flaws improved. I have seen case after case where plastic surgery has helped improve an individual's self–image and added a new vigor or zest to their life.

Today there are many medical and surgical options to improve the outward appearance. Let's examine a few of the less intrusive procedures.

Today one of the most prominent medical treatments for fighting aging skin is Botox. No matter how well skin is preserved and pampered, everyone eventually develops facial wrinkles. Botox is the easiest of all medical options available for removing the lines that accompany aging. It is an extremely quick approach for softening or removing the natural wrinkles that form between the eyes (frown lines), on the forehead, at the sides of the eyes (crow's feet), or at the base of the nose (glabellar frown lines).

Botox is a purified protein toxin that is derived from a

specific form of bacteria. It was originally utilized as a remedy for neck and facial spasms. In the last decade, however, it has been used effectively to remove facial wrinkles.

Each day, the muscles between the eyes (frown lines) or on the outside of the eyes (crow's feet) contract many times. Over time, these muscular contractions create virtual "creases" or wrinkles in the skin. To remove these wrinkles, Botox is injected through a very small needle into the muscles that cause these contractions. The Botox essentially impedes the nerve impulse from reaching these muscles. Gradually, the muscles relax and the facial wrinkles soften or disappear. Patients may experience a slight discomfort when the needle is inserted and the Botox injected, but this only lasts approximately five to seven seconds. The treatment is performed in a physician's office and takes no more than ten to fifteen minutes. In the majority of cases, patients return to their normal routines the same day.

The muscles relax within a few days of the Botox injection, causing wrinkles to either lessen or to disappear completely. The muscles remain in a relaxed state for three to five months. Further treatment is necessary to erase returning wrinkles. After several treatments, the length of time that Botox is effective can increase, sometimes lasting up to eight months.

Botox has been used successfully to diminish facial wrinkles for a number of years and exhibits very few side effects. Although it causes a temporary paralysis of the muscle, it does not affect the nerve, so no numbness in the face occurs. Immediately after the treatment, Botox can spread slightly and possibly lead to a temporary drooping of surrounding muscles. Because of this, patients should avoid rubbing the treated area for 10 to 15 hours following surgery. If drooping does occur, the surrounding muscles typically return to normal within a couple of weeks. In very rare instances, a blood vessel may burst, causing a temporary black and blue area. Patients who are pregnant or have been diagnosed with a neurological disease should refrain from having this procedure performed.[1]

Along with Botox, there is another effective facial procedure called "microdermabrasion." If you have ever noticed how refreshed a stone building looks after a thorough sandblasting, you are on your way to understanding the effects of microdermabrasion. This treatment is basically a buffing process for the outer epidermal layer of the skin, leaving one with smoother, more supple-looking skin. The procedure is relatively new to the United States, but has gained considerable popularity over the past few years.

Microdermabrasion or "microderm" is used to treat sun-damaged skin, unevenly textured skin, fine lines, aging spots, and stretch marks. The procedure involves spraying a fine jet of sand-like crystals onto the skin and, using a highly controlled vacuum, sweeping up the crystals and the top epidermal layer. As microdermabrasion brushes away the damaged cell layers, it also stimulates the skin's production of collagen and helps to maintain the elasticity of the skin. It is a subtle procedure that softens the problem areas of the skin. Many patients return for an additional five to seven treatments over the course of two months to attain a thoroughly refreshed and vibrant appearance.

One of the most favorable aspects of microdermabrasion is that each treatment only takes fifteen to thirty minutes. In fact, microdermabrasion is so convenient that it is often referred to as the "lunchtime face lift." In addition, it requires no anesthesia and is almost completely painless.

Directly following the treatment, the skin typically has a slightly rosy complexion that fades within a day. After microdermabrasion, the skin is often dry and must be properly cleansed and moisturized for several days. In addition, patients should avoid wearing make-up for a day or two after the treatment.

As with any kind of treatment, there are health risks with this procedure. However, since microdermabrasion exfoliates only the external layer of skin, there are rarely serious complications. If a physician is not careful, however, the tiny sand crystals can get in the eyes and cause considerable irritation. Also, those intending to have this procedure performed in a salon need to be aware that there have been cases where the exfoliating crystals have been recycled for multiple patients. These recycled crystals can contain skin toxins from previous patients and can spread serious viruses such as hepatitis. Two weeks prior to the procedure, patients should refrain from tanning or waxing, or having chemical peel or collagen injections performed. Pregnant women should refrain from microdermabrasion altogether.[2]

Another effective cosmetic treatment is the use of collagen. The wearing down of the natural collagen support layer that lies just beneath your skin causes facial lines, deep wrinkles, and creases. External factors, such as exposure to the sun and pollution, and internal conditions, such as the body's natural aging process, also contribute to the wearing down of the collagen layer.

Injectable collagen implant works by supplementing your body's own natural collagen support layer. The liquid collagen is injected via a small needle directly through the wrinkle, skin crease, or skin fold into the support layer just beneath the surface of the skin. The extra support provided by the injectable collagen raises the treated area so that the wrinkle, skin crease, or skin fold disappears. The effect of this treatment is immediately apparent.

Collagen injections are used to treat fine lines, wrinkles, and shallow scars. The areas of the face usually injected are the smile and laugh lines around the mouth, vertical lip lines of the upper and lower lips, and the deep creases between the nose and the outer edges of the mouth. Collagen injections are also used to replace collagen lost from the borders of the upper and lower lips.

The use of any aspirin or other anti-inflammatory medication is prohibited for three days prior to the injections. Some vitamins, such as C and E, have been associated with bruising at the injection site so avoidance of vitamins and herbs for three days before the day of the injections is also recommended. Makeup should not be worn to the office on the day of the injections, but it can be applied immediately afterwards.

When collagen is injected, there is an initial minor sting for a few seconds. Local anesthetic is premixed with the collagen and starts to take effect very soon after the initial injection. Once the injection is complete, there is usually no discomfort. Because the needle is so small and the collagen is premixed with local anesthetic, there is no need for sedation or extra anesthesia. Ice can be applied prior to the injections to numb the skin and to help avoid bruising at the injection sites.

The injections are usually done with the patient in a sitting position, after lightly cleansing the skin with alcohol. There is usually a slight amount of swelling which subsides within 24 hours. You should remain upright for four hours after a collagen treatment. It is further recommended that you do not touch or rub the areas that were injected.

Individuals who have ever had an allergic reaction to injectable collagen products, dietary beef, or lidocaine should not receive collagen injections. These treatments should also be avoided by those with any form of a connective-tissue disorder, such as dermatomyositis or polymyositis.[3] In the near future, pending FDA approval, longer-lasting substances which contain hyaluronic and other microspheres will be available. Artecoll, Perlance, and Restylane have shown tremendous promise, and they are already in use in Europe and Canada.

Now, at this point in the chapter, if you have stopped to examine your face in a mirror and are thinking that you could use a little help in the area of anti-aging, but haven't quite made up your mind to call your doctor to schedule the treatments prescribed above, all is not lost. There are still things you can do to protect your face and skin from the aging process.

Besides the treatments available through a doctor already described, there are also many over-the-counter creams and lotions available on the market. These products, sometimes referred to as a "facial in a bottle," help to prevent the more obvious signs of aging.

Dermatologists suggest that to really prevent the facial skin from aging you must first begin with eating a balanced diet. It is said, "If you are good to the inside, the outside will be good to you." Here are five excellent steps to take:

1. Along with a balanced diet, get eight hours of sleep each night and think positive thoughts. Remember, if you are going to get wrinkles, get the ones that accompany a smile rather than a frown.

2. Drink eight glasses of water a day. Adequate hydration of the body is important for all the body's functions.

3. Take a multivitamin and the antioxidants vitamin E and vitamin C. Recent scientific evidence suggests that when vitamin E (400 units) and vitamin C (250mg-500mg) are taken orally, they may help remove the free radicals that cause skin damage from sun exposure.

4. Moisturize the skin. The skin—like shoe leather—will become dried out if not treated properly. Rehydrate the skin daily with a moisturizer. Not all people require a moisturizer.

5. Vitamin C creams and lotions increase collagen production and reduce the damaging effects of the sun. Not all topical vitamin C creams will improve the skin. Only those preparations with stable forms of L-ascorbic acid (vitamin C) are beneficial.

Some of the external creams are often referred to as "plastic surgery in a bottle" due to the success rate in helping women look younger. Look for products that contain substances like carnosine, aminoguanadine, alpha lipoic acid, DMAE, tocotrienols, slenomethoine, ascorbyl palmitate, COQ-10, and Pyruvate. These are not only powerful antioxidants, but in the case of Pyruvate, prevent the formation of free radicals.

In addition, carnosine, lipoic acid, and aminoguanadine, break glycation products that cause crosslinking and chronic inflammation that wrinkles and ages the skin. Some recent advances have also led to oral drinks and supplements that specifically increase collagen production, which is the foundation of the skin, therefore resolving lines, wrinkles and age spots.

I also want to emphasize that your eating habits affect the state of your skin. A healthy diet will improve all aspects of your life, including your external appearance. I can assure you that face and eyelid lifts and liposuction can literally be prolonged by regulating diet and stress. It's also important to limit caffeine intake and to make sure you drink at least eight glasses of water each day. (*For a more detailed description of diet and the effects of stress, see the chapters entitled* "An Apple a Day..." *and* "STRESS: Can't Live With (Too Much of) It & Can't Live Without (Any of) It.")

It is also important to remember that sun is dangerous to the skin. Noel Coward said that only "mad dogs and Englishmen go out in the midday sun." Whereas, I may not have the statistics to back up Mr. Coward's claim, I certainly have the data to show that those who repeatedly expose unprotected skin to the sun are practically guaranteeing future skin problems.

The power of the sun to damage our skin is sometimes underestimated. Ultraviolet radiation injures the cells that produce elastin and collagen fibers, causing wrinkles. It also over-stimulates pigment cells, creating irregular coloring, including the brown blotches, erroneously called liver spots, that appear on faces, forearms, and hands.

The damaging effects of sunlight on skin go far beyond wrinkling, toughening, and discoloring. Sun exposure accounts for roughly 90 percent of skin cancer and is considered one of the major causes of cataracts. Repeated exposure to ultraviolet radiation damages the skin cells' genetic material. As the earth's ozone layer thins, the sun's rays, which penetrate clouds, are becoming more intense and more dangerous.

You can protect yourself by always using a sunscreen with a sun protection factor (SPF) of at least 15. To determine how long you should stay out in the sun, multiply the SPF listed on sunscreen by the length of time it takes your unprotected skin to burn. If you are fair, you probably start to redden after 12 minutes. Multiplying 12 (minutes to redden) by 15 (SPF) gives you 180 minutes—or three hours—to stay safely outdoors wearing a liberal amount of sunscreen on all exposed skin. It's important to reapply sunscreen after swimming or perspiring heavily. Remember, however, that reapplication doesn't allow you to stay out longer, it simply restores the protection you had when you first put on sunscreen.

The SPF factor refers to protection against only one kind of ultraviolet rays, those called UBA. UVA rays also cause skin damage. Only sunscreens labeled "broad spectrum" give full UVA and UVB protection. Look for the ingredient Parsol 1789 (avobenzone), which has been proven effective against UVA.

If your skin is sensitive to chemical sunscreens, use titanium dioxide ointment, which blocks ultraviolet rays by reflecting sunlight. For particularly sensitive areas, such as the nose, the tips of the ears, or the top of a bald head, use titanium dioxide ointment or another sun block such as zinc oxide. Also, remember to cover the skin with opaque clothing (denim is good) that is dry (sun can penetrate a wet T-shirt). A wide-brimmed hat can protect your face and eyes from direct sunlight but not from reflected light bouncing off sand, snow, or water; so always wear appropriate sunglasses, too.

Sun strength varies with the season and time of day. Many of my colleagues suggest staying indoors between 11 a. m. and 3 p.m. in summer. Elevation and distance from the equator are also important. Shorten your daily sun time in the tropics and in the mountains.

You should also be aware that certain medications (some antibiotics, for example) make your skin more sun sensitive. Check with your own doctor about any drugs you are taking.[4]

Finally, you need to remember that cigarettes are harmful. Former U.S. Surgeon General C. Everett Koop M.D has declared: "Cigarettes are the most important health risk in this country, responsible for more premature deaths and disability than any other known agent." Research has shown that quitting now will give you a younger heart and cardiovascular system, and, because smoking also increases the risk of lung cancer 10 to 25 times, stopping now will remove you from these high-risk groups. But, if the threat of a terminal illness isn't enough to get a smoker to quit, Dr. Koop could add that smoking ruins your skin, too.

Although the tobacco industry spends billions of dollars promoting smoking as being glamorous, twenty years of epidemiological research has concluded that smokers typically suffer enhanced facial aging and skin wrinkling termed "smoker's face."

As early as 1856, the presence of skin changes in cigarette smokers was noted. Such changes include increased wrinkling, a slightly reddened or orange complexion, mild puffiness, and gauntness. "Smoker's face" is also characterized by elastotic changes—the breakdown of the elastic fibers of the skin which give rise to yellow irregularly thickened skin.

Research has also found that women's skin seems to be more affected by the adverse effects of smoking than men's, and that wrinkling increases with the duration and amount of smoking, which is linked to the chemicals within tobacco.

Cigarette smoke is capable of damaging collagen and elastin in lung tissue and may cause elastotic changes in the skin of smokers by similar mechanisms. It is conceivable that the clinical changes in smokers' skin, including the gray-tinted skin and the prominent wrinkling, may be due to this increase in elastotic material. Other studies have noted that the skin of a smoker contains less water, possibly accounting for some of these clinical changes. Since nicotine does have a diuretic effect on the body, it would follow that the moisture content of a smoker's skin would be lessened.

The vascular structure of the skin may also play a role in elastotic changes. "The skin's vascular structure is constricted by acute and long-term smoking. The resulting decrease in blood flow may induce local skin irritation and carry more toxic substances to these tissues. (Or, in other words) the skin is weakened—and it wrinkles," explains dermatologist Alan S. Boyd, MD.

Clinically, aggravation of elastosis has been described in persons subjected to heat in the workplace—including bakers, firemen and engineers. Studies have noted glass blowers have symptoms of severe skin aging even in early adulthood. Increased skin elastosis is not a result of slowed degradation of existing elastic fibers, but rather from the exaggerated elastin produced by repeated blasts of heat. Continuing research concludes that the presence of a continuous source of heat, such as a lit cigarette, may have promoted the increased elastosis found in the skin of smokers.

The effects of smoking and sun damage may be synergistic. Since regular sunscreen use will fight the effects of UV rays, the recommendation that smokers use sunscreens may prevent some of the damage. However, until sunscreens contain materials to reflect heat absorption, the damaging chemical and thermal effects of smoking will continue.

The best prevention against "smoker's face" is to stop smoking. Increasing public awareness of the association between smoking and wrinkles could be just the added incentive some individuals need to throw their cigarettes away for good. While it can be difficult to realistically grasp how cigarettes damage the tissue of the lungs, one look in a well-lighted mirror may provide all the proof needed to see how cigarettes damage the skin.[5]

Josh Billings once remarked that "In youth we run into difficulties, in old age difficulties run into us." Whereas there is no current research that leads me to believe aging will become obsolete, there are certainly products, procedures, and lifestyle changes that can help each of us better weather or avoid old age difficulties. The research is on-going, the products are being developed, and the youthful possibilities are endless.

Forever Facts:
   We are judged by our appearance.
   Protect yourself from the sun.
   Stop smoking today.
   Check with a plastic surgeon on the best options for putting your best face forward.

Endnotes:

1. Information on Botox derived from Dimitry Khasak, M.D., Board-Certified Dermatologist and a member of the Intense Pulsed Light Education Institute, the American Academy of Dermatology, and the National Psoriasis Foundation.

2. Information on Microdermabrasion derived from Dimitry Khasak, M.D., Board-Certified Dermatologist and a member of the Intense Pulsed Light Education Institute, the American Academy of Dermatology, and the National Psoriasis Foundation.

3. Information on collagen injections derived from Lewis Self, M.D.

4. Information on effects of sun on skin derived from Doctor's Report, "Live Longer/Live Better," *Reader's Digest.*

5. Information on the effects of smoking on the skin derived from dermatologist Alan S. Boyd, MD, Department of Dermatology, Vanderbilt University,"Cigarette Smoking-Associated Elastotic Changes in the Skin," *Journal of the American Academy of Dermatology,* July 1999.

*"We have a lot of anxieties, and one cancels out
another very often."*
—*Winston Churchill*

STRESS: Can't Live With (Too Much of) It And Can't Live Without (Any of) It

Have you ever tried juggling? Professional jugglers seem to easily keep balls, plates, jagged knives, burning torches, and a variety of other objects whirling effortlessly in the air. If you are a novice giving juggling a try, however, you will find it is much more difficult than it looks. To be a successful juggler, you have to maintain a tension and constant rhythm to keep the objects moving. If you jerk or move too quickly or too slowly, the tension and rhythm are broken. Control of the whirling objects is lost, and you better look out for flying debris.

In the hectic, fast-paced rhythm of life today, juggling is required. The tension needed to keep things up in the air is stress, an unavoidable part of life. To a certain degree, however, stress is not necessarily negative. It can be a motivator, can keep you "on your toes," and can keep things moving.

Jeff Herring, a licensed marriage and family therapist and clinical hypnotherapist, shares a universal law about stress. He reports, "Believe it or not we all need a little stress in our lives. Too little and there is not motivation for change. Too much and we begin to shut down and get overwhelmed. It is important to know your optimal level of stress and then do all the necessary things to keep your stress level in balance." One of the major causes of stress is having too much to do and being pulled in too many directions at one time.

Oftentimes you can begin to feel like you are on a treadmill with no way to get off. If and when this happens, it is time to STOP and take a look at where you are going. Review your calendar, go over your commitments, and ask yourself a few questions. Are all the commitments absolutely necessary? Is there anything that can be postponed or even eliminated? What can be delegated? Of course there are certain responsibilities that you must take care of, but give yourself at least 15 to 30 minutes a day JUST FOR YOU. If you don't, then the stress levels become out of balance and can be damaging to your health.

After listening to tapes of studies done a number of years ago, I found that the expected lifespan for a doctor was then 58 years old. The reason was not exposure to germs or too much radiation from x-rays. The reason for the low life expectancy was due to stressors associated with the occupation.

As early as the 1930s, Hans Seyle found a direct connection between your reaction to stressors (traffic jams, financial problems, and personality conflicts) and your health.

It is not surprising that today in our more hectic lifestyle, the connection between stressors and health problems continues to prove true. According to a June 14, 1999 article in *Newsweek* magazine, the chances of catching a cold increase the longer people experience work or interpersonal stress, and men, who say they are highly stressed, are more likely to have heart attacks and strokes.

In a 1998 study, Psychologist Sheldon Cohen of Carnegie Mellon University found it's not the big incidents like your teenager's car accident or favorite uncle's death that cause the most stress. It's the small but ongoing conflicts that increase the odds of stress-related illness by three to five times.

Stress can be real or imagined. Even though stress is an inevitable part of daily life, being "stressed out" doesn't have to be. The problem with stressors is that once they are ignited, the fire of your neurological and hormonal responses can't be stopped. When you can't fight or flee, the stressors develop physical responses in your body to deal with the stress.

Dr. Julian Whitaker, M.D. suggests we all need to have an outlet for stress. He believes: "If we can't vent our emotions in a healthy way, we may completely deplete ourselves by turning all that negative energy inward. This results in physical symptoms such as stomachaches, headaches, and even heart palpitations. Clearly, we need to manage and modulate our emotional and physical reactions through positive action. If you're having a tough day at home with the kids or if a coworker angers you, don't just sit back and simmer. When you feel anxious and keyed up, acknowledge that you're under stress and then do something to alleviate it."

One of the best things to do when you are "stressed to the max" is to move your body. Exercise helps deplete the circulating stress hormones so you can calm down faster. Even if you don't have the time or inclination for a full workout, a brisk five- or ten-minute walk will release tension and help you unwind.

If you can't exercise, listening to music is a great stress releaser. Soothing songs work great, as well as jazzy, catchy tunes you can sing along with.

I have found another simple way of eliminating stress is to stop thinking of all that is wrong and focus on the good things in my life. When I center my thoughts on my wife, my daughter, kind friends, supportive coworkers, and the good I can do in the world, I feel less stressed. I think it's essential to take some time during the day to remind yourself of what is good in your life. You might even make a list of your blessings so that any time you find yourself focusing solely on the negative, you can balance it with positive thoughts of gratitude.

Not all stress is set in the moment or related to a bad day. Some sources of stress are long-term and on-going. Here are nine suggested steps you can take to eradicate this destructive stress from your life.

Step 1—Resolve Grudges

When a woman, who had lived to be 101 years old, was asked to share the secret of her long life, she replied, "I learned to forget." She explained that she meant she learned to forget, and thereby forgive, all the wrongs, slights, criticisms, and conflicts that could have sapped her energy.

Researchers have confirmed this woman's secret to a long life. They have found the best way to become stress resistant and improve quality of life is to resolve grudges and prevent new ones from forming.

"Oh yeah?" (You may be thinking to yourself.) "That's easy for you to say." Skepticism is justified here. Shakespeare said, "It were easier to tell twenty men what was good to be done than to be one of the twenty to follow mine instruction." It is much easier to talk about resolving grudges than to do it. But the following suggestions might help.

- Evaluate the true impact of the damage done by an offending person. Has someone died, lost a limb, or is living on the streets with nothing to eat as a result of this person's behavior? Try to put things into perspective.

- Resolve to take responsibility for only what YOU can control. Let go of your efforts to try and change the person against whom you harbor a grudge. You can choose to let this individual continue to damage your life, or you can move beyond it.

- Identify one positive thing that came as a result of the offender's behavior. Perhaps you are a smarter, stronger, or better person today from having to deal with this individual.

Step 2—Get More Rest

Sleep deprivation causes 100,000 automobile accidents per year. The majority of all Americans only get 6.7 hours of sleep per night, despite the fact that adults need 8 to 10 hours, and teenagers require an average of 9 hours and 15 minutes. The importance of adequate sleep on performance is validated in a study of 3,100 Rhode Island students. The study found that, on average, those getting A's and B's got 35 minutes more sleep a night than those who made C's and D's.

At this point, you may be asking yourself, "How, in my already overburdened, stressed-out life, do I find the time to get more sleep?!" In an article entitled, "Stress Solving Strategies," by Laura Benjamin, she suggests that one of the most important things we can do is maintain a consistent sleep schedule, even on vacation and weekends. Ms. Benjamin affirms that sleep deprivation impacts the aging process. She says that you can't undo damage from lack of sleep by trying to "catch up."

Begin now to plan on getting the right amount of sleep. Try to go to bed near the same time every night. If it is difficult to turn your thoughts off, there are several nutritional sleep aids you can try.

Melatonin, a natural hormone known for its ability to regulate sleep cycles, is a veritable cure for insomnia for many people. Produced in the pineal gland, a pea-sized structure embedded deep in the brain, melatonin controls the body's circadian rhythm, which informs us when it's time to sleep and to awaken. Melatonin is also a potent antioxidant and has been shown in animal studies to significantly extend life and reverse many of the telltale signs of aging.

Melatonin is at its peak level in childhood, drops during adolescence when other hormones kick in, and continues to decrease as you age. By sixty, our pineal gland is producing half the amount of melatonin it did when we were twenty.

Taking tiny doses of melatonin supplements at nighttime can shorten the amount of time it takes to fall asleep and restore normal sleep cycles. Another benefit of melatonin is that, unlike sleeping pills, it is not addictive.

Step 3—Prioritize

Often we create our own stress. We take on too many things because we have a hard time saying, "No!" Our time is stretched between home, work, and community. Today in our fast-paced world, the term "multi-tasking" has become elevated to heroic proportions.

Dr. Richard A. Swenson, in his book *Margin*, states we are reaching our saturation point by trying to do just "one more thing" throughout the day. The more we try to cram in, the more mistakes we make, the less time we truly listen to each other (because we're trying to type an e-mail or answer a call at the same time), and, consequently, the more stressed we become. Dr. Swenson suggests, "Rather than trying to do one more thing, consider eliminating those tasks and appointments that are not critical and do not give you the biggest 'bang for the buck'." In other words, set your priorities and eliminate the non-essentials.

Step 4—Change Word Usage

Several years ago, a popular woman's magazine came out with an article on how to relieve stress. One of the suggested ways was quite simple, but, if put into effect, was estimated to reduce your stress level by 35 percent. The suggestion was to take 3 very stressful phrases out of your vocabulary and replace them with 3 positive ones. The phrases to get rid of are: "I *have to, I should*," and "I *can't*." This suggestion may seem very simple, but think about it. What kind of emotional response do you have when you use those 3 phrases? Now think of how you feel when you say, "I *could, I want* to," or "I *can*." What a difference! The first three phrases make us feel acted upon by outside sources, while the last three phrases make us feel in control of what we do. That feeling of being in control is a great stress reducer.

There is another word that might be good to include in your stress-reducing vocabulary. Psychologists have done studies and found that the word, "interesting," is the only word in the English language to *not* provoke an emotional response. So, as you are driving in traffic and are cut off by a mentally deficient road hog, if you can say to yourself, "That was an *interesting* maneuver," rather than commenting on the driver's ancestry, mental competence, and obvious shady maneuvers in securing a driver's license, it will diffuse your feelings of stress and make you feel more relaxed and in control of the situation.

Step 5—Learn to Let Go of Things Out of Your Control

A man, who has experienced much of the harshness of life, was a successful young boxer during his high school years, becoming Idaho's State Champion. When interviewed, he was asked how he could go into the boxing ring and always come out without mussing his hair. His answer has application to stressful situations in life.

The boxer said, "I had to learn to let go of things out of my control. I had trained, and studied everything I could about the sport, and kept abreast of my opponent, his moves, his short-comings, etc. I did everything I could to prepare. I accepted the challenge. But when I stepped into the ring, I told myself, 'Let go. You know what to do. Don't panic. Just put out your best shot. Don't worry about the outcome. There will always be other fights.'"

This great man has felt many of the "blows" in life. When they came, however, he took his own advice. He accepted the challenge, didn't panic, and gave it his best "punch."

Step 6—Go On a Diet from the Media

Don't immerse yourself in all the headlines and watch every news broadcast. Be alert, learn what you need to know in order to protect yourself and your children, and find out ways to help people who are in need. But, don't listen to all the arguing, debating, and doomsday prognosticators on TV and radio stations. A continual diet of political discussions alone can raise your blood pressure and leave you feeling downhearted. Some psychologists suggest that leaving the television and radio turned off and limiting your newspaper exposure can prevent the stress that comes from outside concerns. Take the advice of a woman who lived to be 122 years old: "If you can't do anything about it, don't worry about it."

Step 7—Utilize Relaxation Techniques

Two great ways to unwind and relax that I would recommend are yoga and aromatherapy. Yoga helps to put things in perspective. The key is that this meditative, relaxing technique centers on breathing. Try the following:

- Sitting quietly with your hands in your lap or gently resting beside you, close your eyes and breathe lightly and normally.
- Listen as the air passes down into your lungs through your nostrils and then softly up and out. The breath should be gentle and easy. As your breathing relaxes, try

making it a little lighter. If you begin to feel short of breath, breathe in a bit.

- Allow your body to dictate what air you need, concentrating on the internal sounds and sensations of air moving in, through, and out of your body. Do this for ten to twenty minutes.

By paying attention to your breathing, you will sink deeper and deeper into a state of relaxation, thus quieting your mind. You will feel calm and yet refreshed, and ready to face the rest of your day.

Sometimes the answer to stress may be right under your nose—literally. Growing in popularity by leaps and bounds, aromatherapy utilizes the power of scent to soothe, relax, and heal. Nearly two thousand years ago, Hippocrates, the father of modern medicine, noted that "the way to health is to have an aromatic bath and a scented massage every day." Since ancient times, healers have used the essential oils from spices and herbs to treat various illnesses of the body and the mind.

Today, studies have documented the power of essential oils to relax and recharge the body and mind. Aromatic oils are sold in thousands of herb shops and department stores around the country, with dozens of oils to choose from. Generally, you can use one oil at a time or combine several. Most herb shops will let you sample several oils so that you can custom design your own aromatherapy treatment. Remember that a little oil goes a long way. You only need a few drops to experience the full benefit of aromatherapy.

Remember this is *aroma* therapy. The oils are to be inhaled and NOT ingested. Don't inhale an essential oil directly from the bottle because the scent may be too strong and could be irritating. Instead, boil one quart of water and add ten drops of oil. Inhale the steam.

You can also bathe in the oils. Add five to ten drops of essential oil to a warm bath. Relax in the tub for at least fifteen minutes and let your stress go down the drain.

Two oils found especially effective in relieving stress are chamomile and citrus.

Chamomile oil can soothe the spirit and is especially helpful when you are tense or irritable. You might even want to keep a bottle of this in your desk at work, along with a container for hot water!

Citrus oil (particularly grapefruit and orange) will help lift you out of the blues. In one Japanese study, after using citrus aromatherapy for four to eleven weeks, patients, who had been taking antidepressants daily, were able to cut back or even eliminate their medication.

Step 8—Let in the Light

One simple solution for relieving stress is to pull up the shades and let in the sunshine. Sunlight stimulates your brain and gives you a natural lift. This is a safe way to take advantage of sunlight without exposing your skin to ultraviolet rays.

You might also try using full-spectrum lights. Put these lights in one or two rooms at home or at work where you spend the most time. You don't even have to buy new fixtures.

Go out in the sun. Winter doesn't offer as many sunny days as warmer seasons, but taking even brief walks, warmly dressed, out in the weaker rays of winter sunshine will lift you out of the "winter blues."

Step 9—Reach Out to Pets, Plants, and People

It has been proven that those who have pets live longer. The unconditional acceptance of a pet is soothing to the psyche.

Growing things is a good stress reliever, as well. Gardening combines physical activity, outward focus, and the fun that comes from watching plants grow. And, if you need a listening ear, talk to your plants. Some research suggests plants grow better if they are talked to in a kind voice.

Reach out to people. We all need people, whether we think we do or not. We learn from others, gain strength from others, and feel better about life by associating with others. Whether it is saying hello to the mailman or smiling at someone you meet going into a grocery store, connecting with people will lower your stress ratio.

Life *is* a juggling act, and stress is certainly a byproduct. No matter how hard we try, we can't escape all stress. I believe the key, however, is not to eliminate stress, but rather learn to control stress, and not allow it to control you.

Forever Facts:

Eat a proper diet. Good fuel always helps the body function better.

Be patient with yourself. You're human. Don't hold yourself to an impossible standard.

Express your feelings to others calmly. Raising your voice and getting angry are non-productive.

Develop your creative side through poetry, writing, music, or dance. Creative expression can be an outlet for stressful feelings and help you feel good about you.

Enjoy your friendships. Remember that to have friends, you need to be one. And, remember to be a good friend to yourself.

Keep a positive outlook on life. The more negative you are, the more hopeless your mindset.

Keep a journal. Psychologists have found this to be a very therapeutic, cathartic exercise.

"The bad news is time flies. The good news is you are the pilot."
—H. Jackson Brown

Utilizing the Principle of Balance

Have you ever sat in the stands under the circus big top, watching the tightrope walker high above your head? Holding your breath, you keep tabs on the circus performer's progress across the narrow wire. When he reaches safety on the other side, you barely have time to catch a breath before another performer takes his place, heading back into harm's way. This performer stretches your nerves even tighter with some gravity-defying feat on the tightrope wire, like jumping rope, balancing on a chair, or climbing on top of someone's shoulders. Your heart pounds as you anxiously gaze upward, expecting any minute for the worst to happen. But, it rarely does, because the tightrope walker understands the principle of balance. He knows how to shift his weight and the objects he works with as he climbs, moves, and jumps on that wire in order to maintain perfect balance and avoid a mishap.

Whether or not we are still nursing a childhood fantasy to run away and join the circus, there is a life lesson to be learned under the big top. I believe that all of us need to understand and utilize the principle of balance in our lives. We need to make sure that our time and energy is balanced among the important areas of our lives in order to keep our mental, emotional, spiritual, and social health intact.

The following are considered the four basic human needs. These are areas of our lives where we need to maintain and utilize the principle of balance.

Physical Needs

A human being has a physical need for things, such as food, clothing, shelter, and economic security. To ensure we have these physical necessities, work is a requisite. Each of us needs to be gainfully employed in order to meet our financial requirements. If we are lucky, our life's work is not just a requirement or a necessity, but it gives us a sense of purpose, of direction, and of accomplishment. Ulysses S. Grant once said, "Labor disgraces no man, but occasionally men disgrace labor." Work, at its very best, should bring a feeling of satisfaction for a job well done. Sometimes, however, it is easy to overdose on work—to become a workaholic. If we prefer working overtime at the office instead of being at home with family or friends, our life is out of balance. We need to remember Don Herold's advice: "Work is the greatest thing in the world, so we should always save some of it for tomorrow."

Family and Friends

Each of us has a social need to relate to other people: to belong, to love, and to be loved. The family is the basic unit of society. A family that functions well is not only a blessing to society, but a blessing to the members of that family as well. My relationship with my parents, grandmother, and other family members has been a tremendous help to me throughout my life. Love and respect were constants in our familial interactions, and I knew my family cared for me and would always be there to support and advise me.

Ideally, the family is where we receive the kind of balanced social support and closeness we need to sustain us, especially when we are experiencing tough times. Good family life takes time and care to develop, but is certainly worth the effort.

Friends also fulfill an important social need and help keep our lives in balance. Psychologists have discovered that when people start struggling with depression or have emotional or mental problems, one of their instinctive reactions is to shut themselves off from people. Unfortunately, this is one of the worst things they can do. Spending time with friends and interacting with others helps limit introspection and broadens our horizons.

A woman who struggled with an anxiety disorder was invited to a small dinner party with friends. She did not want to go. However, concerned about offending her hostess, a good friend, she got dressed up and forced herself to attend the party. On the way over, she felt extremely anxious and was fighting a sensation of "dread." Once she got involved in the accepting and friendly environment of the party, however, she had a great time. She got so enmeshed in a game the group was playing that she scored the final points, snatching victory for her team. Driving home from the party, she felt relaxed, calm, and balanced.

In the case of friendship, we might want to remember Samuel Johnson's advice: "If a man does not make new acquaintances as he advances through life, he will soon find himself left alone. One should keep his friendships in constant repair."

Self

A life is also out of balance if we don't have time for ourselves. We need time for contemplation, for deep thinking. Each of us has a mental need to develop, grow, and to set goals to secure achievement. There is something in each of us that wants to capture a corner of immortality by bequeathing something to the next generation. It's important for us to organize ourselves and our lives so that we are personally able to give something back.

George Bernard Shaw says: "This is the true joy of

life...being used for a purpose recognized by yourself as a mighty one...being a force of Nature instead of a feverish, selfish, little clod of ailments and grievances, complaining that the world will not devote itself to making you happy...I am of the opinion that my life belongs to the whole community. As long as I live, it is my privilege to do for it whatever I can. I want to be thoroughly used up when I die. For the harder I work, the more I live. I rejoice in life for its own sake. Life is no brief candle to me. It's a sort of splendid torch which I've to hold up for the moment, and I want to make it burn as brightly as possible before handing it on to future generations."

A life that is a "splendid torch" is a life in balance where we know ourselves and feel content with who we are and what we have accomplished.

God

Each of us has a spiritual need for a sense of meaning, of purpose, and of personal congruence in our lives. There is a part in each of us that yearns to live for a higher purpose than self.

September 11, 2001 is a day that is imprinted upon the minds of millions of people. Watching the planes crash into the World Trade Center and the Pentagon was like viewing a scene from a horror film. In the aftermath of this tragedy, it was reassuring to note where comfort was sought. Congress gathered on the steps of the Capitol Building to sing "God Bless America." The President declared a "National Day of Prayer." Attendance at churches and synagogues dramatically increased as Americans sought for the comfort and peace that comes from acknowledgment of a Higher Power.

There is a beautiful hymn written by Emma Lou Thayne entitled "Where Can I Turn for Peace?" It reads:

Where can I turn for peace? Where is my solace?
When other sources cease to make me whole?
When with a wounded heart, anger, or malice,
I draw myself apart, searching my soul?
Where, when my aching grows, Where, when I languish,
Where, in my need to know, where can I run?
Where is the quiet hand to calm my anguish?
Who, who can understand? He, only One.

This spiritual fulfillment and meaning to life brings a balance and a wholeness to our existence. My mother never failed to reiterate to us, "Always remember God."

Attending to the four basic needs in your life and utilizing the principle of balance takes time. Try the following four suggestions to free up time and make life a little easier for yourself.

SIMPLIFY—Do you ever feel that life is too busy—too complex? Perhaps a little simplification can help you find the time you never seem to have for things like spending time with the family or even reading the newspaper. Too many of us fill our time with projects and tasks that can be delegated or discarded all together. We are often conditioned to thinking that the more we do, the greater will be our success. Often this mindset keeps us off-balance and takes time away from those we love and who need us most. An effective balancing measure is to make sure that the *majority* of our time is not spent on the things that matter *least*.

SAY NO—When you are asked to do something that will add more pressure or take you away from those most important to you, remember Nancy Reagan's advice to "Just say NO!" You can kindly and politely thank the person asking you and then firmly say, "No." Remember you do not have to make excuses for the reason you aren't able to give assistance. If you are afraid of offending, there are ways of verbalizing "No" very clearly without actually saying the word. For instance, you might say:

> "Thank you for asking, perhaps another time."
>
> "Your confidence in me is appreciated.
>
> Why don't you put me down for another time."
>
> "It was so kind of you to think of me.
>
> I hope you'll ask me again when my schedule is a little freer."

DELEGATE—Ask others to help out. Co-workers, family, and friends are great sources of support. Don't try to be Superman or Superwoman. It helps to have others' assistance, and it helps for others to be involved. You don't have to do everything or carry the burdens of the world on your shoulders alone. Remember John Ruskin's assertion: "Every great man is always being helped by everybody; for his gift is to get good out of all things and all persons."

DON'T SAY "I DON'T HAVE TIME"—The more you tell yourself, "I don't have the time...," the more pressure you feel. Sometimes you just need a reminder to take stock of yourself to use the time you have more wisely. It's important to prioritize and make sure your time is being used on the significant things in your life.

Imagine you have in front of you a gallon bucket. On one side of the bucket you have a stack of large stones. On the other side you have a pile of sand. If you scoop up enough sand to fill the bucket halfway full and then try to pile the stones on top, you will soon run out of room. However, if you pile the stones in first and then drizzle in the sand, the bucket will hold much more.

The same thing is true with our lives. After we take care of our top priorities, then it's easier to work in time for the things of lesser importance.

The preceding ideas, if followed, can help us to lead a more balanced life. I want to emphasize that the principle of balance in human existence does not spontaneously operate. We need to manually put it into effect.

Forever Facts:

Check over your week's schedule. Is your time balanced between the four basic human needs?

Take time to socialize. Don't wait for friends to call you. Call them and offer an invitation.

Socializing doesn't have to be expensive or elaborate. Pop some popcorn, rent a movie, and call some friends.

Remember that with family life QUALITY of time never does replace QUANTITY.

Spending time on "you" is a prerequisite not an elective.

If difficult for you, practice saying "No" in the mirror until it becomes easier.

Sometimes we won't delegate because we don't want to give up control.

"The unfortunate thing about this world is that the good habits are much easier to give up than the bad ones."
—W. Somerset Maugham

Letting the Best of You Emerge

A story is told of a talented art student who had enrolled in a sculpturing class. Each student in the class had been given a block of clay, along with the date when their first sculpture was due. This particular student took the clay block home and immediately began to manipulate and work the clay, removing a piece of clay from one section and building up and smoothing another. After working for some time, he stepped back and looked at his "work." It looked like a "glob" of clay. For several days, he started over again and again, but, each time, the result was a "glob." Sometimes it was a smaller glob, a bigger glob, a smoother glob, or a rougher glob, but, on each and every occasion, the clay continued to look like a "glob." As the due date loomed closer, the student made an appointment with his professor, seeking additional guidance, hoping to keep from flunking the class. Meeting with his professor, the student explained his problem. The professor said that whenever he was working on a sculpture, before he ever touched the medium, whether it was a block of clay, wood, or stone, he would set the block in a space where he would see it often. Each day he would look at the medium, examine its texture, and think about it. He would try to visualize the beautiful piece contained within that block. It was only after he had the final work clearly in his mind, that he began to sculpt. At that point, it was just a matter of removing the excess and allowing the beautiful image to emerge.

The professor's advice also has application for the medium of life. For those who are trying to create something beautiful, long lasting, and valuable from this earthly experience, it is helpful to follow the professor's format of creation. It is meaningful to examine your life and carefully think about it. It is important to clearly visualize what you want the end result of your life to be. Then, after making sure you have your final "work" clearly in mind, you need to ask yourself what things are excess that need to be removed to allow the best of you to emerge.

This is the time for honesty. What in your life needs removing or fixing? Grab a pad and pencil. Make a list of all the things in your life that you don't like about yourself, or elements in your left that you'd like to change. Review your list and make sure it is realistic. Remember your list should consist of things you *can* change. It might be helpful to keep in mind the well-known "Serenity Prayer":

> "God,
> Grant me the Serenity
> To accept the things I cannot change,
> The Courage to change the things I can,
> And the Wisdom to know the difference."

Keeping this advice in mind, begin working on the things you can change. You should list those habits, those learned patterns of action you've developed, that need to be cut away, that are marring the final product of what you want to become. It is easy to fall into the trap of allowing a negative habit to dominate your life, causing you to feel trapped. Humans are creatures of habits and some of those habits are good, but, sad to say, some of them aren't.

The brain can store information about how to do routine

activities, and then use that information whenever needed without having to think about it purposely. Doing the same thing every day the same way impresses it in your mind and can make an action almost an automated response. Much of what you do every day is routine or, in other words, habit-forming. Some of these habits make life a little easier, like when you automatically take a shower or brush your teeth. But, unfortunately, while you are registering all these helpful experiences, it is oftentimes easy to develop bad habits, unwise patterns of doing things the wrong way.

I suggest that some common negative habits that many people fight are overeating, excessive television watching, smoking, drinking too much, living off fast food, procrastinating, etc. No one is completely free of bad habits. And, sadly, behaviors can become habits so easily that you don't realize it is a habit, until is has taken control of you.

The problem with bad habits is that they are things that obscure your best. Bad habits can affect your health, limiting the things you are able to do. Bad habits lessen your cognitive function, slowing memory and thinking processes. Bad habits can lower your self-esteem, leading to a feeling of weakness that a "thing" is in control of your life, rather than you.

Bad habits happen, but they can be broken, enabling you to live a better life. Benjamin Franklin gives this encouragement: "Each year, one vicious habit rooted out, in time ought to make the worst man good."

So, realizing the possibilities and that you are in control of your life, I would like to suggest the following habit-breaking steps.

Step One—Have a Desire to Change

You must first *desire* to change. It is the nature of human beings to resist change. You can't overcome a bad habit unless you really want to change. You must be serious before you will be motivated to take the necessary steps.

Step Two—Recognition of Triggers

Recognize when you are developing a bad habit. Think back and keep a record of what seems to trigger it. Are you alone when indulging in this bad habit? Are there certain friends that encourage you? How often do you repeat it? Don't place the blame on someone else. Remember it is *your* habit. However, if someone may be influencing you to participate in negative behaviors, you may need to stay away from that person and get some new friends.

If your spouse or children encourage something negative, like fast food eating, have a family meeting, explain to them how you feel, and ask for their support. It is often helpful to use "I" messages when asking for help in matters like this. For instance, you can say something like, "When you *do* this, I *feel* this..." Experts say that "I" messages get your point across without pointing the finger of blame.

Step Three—Replace Bad Habits with Good Ones

Replace a bad habit with a positive behavior. Herbert W. Armstrong, the author of *The Plain Truth*, uses this analogy. He says the best way to get air out of a glass or jar is to put something else, such as water, in to force the air out. It is the same with bad habits. To force them out of your life, you must replace them with something good.

For instance, if you are a TV-aholic, turn off the TV, and *DO* something. Go for a walk, visit a friend, swing on the front porch, play with a pet, go to the library, or find a good book, etc. Do something that takes your attention away the negative behavior, investing your time into something more positive.

Step Four—Stop Immediately

Stop a habit immediately. Completely halting the negative behavior *immediately* is by far the most effective method of breaking a bad habit. For example, tapering off the amount you smoke doesn't work for most smokers.

Selecting a date on the calendar when you will smoke your last cigarette and then stopping on that day has been found to be more successful in long-term change. Make sure your commitment is a firm one.

Step Five—No Excuses

Don't make excuses. Our habits actually program us to resist change. Once a habit is ingrained, it can become invisible to the conscious mind, and we try to ignore it or rationalize it away. Refuse to think, "I can't change. I'm just that way. Nobody's perfect." Thoughts like that will only reinforce the chains that the habit has on you.

Step Six—Be Positive

Be positive and enthusiastic. Don't get discouraged. It won't be easy, and sometimes you might slip backwards. The important thing is to just keep working on it. Be positive about your decision to gain more control of your life. Remember you're heading for success. Stick with it.

Step Seven—You've Got to Have Faith

Have faith in yourself. Realize that you have the power to change. You are in control of You. Make up your mind and GO FOR IT!

So . . . what are you waiting for? Go on! Get started. Break a bad habit. Even by taking a small step, you are starting a new pattern. Breaking even one bad habit can give you a feeling of satisfaction and encouragement as nothing else will. Keep it up and chip away at all the negative excess in your life, allowing the best of you to emerge. The rewards, I can assure you, will be well worth the effort.

<u>Forever Facts:</u>

You have the power of control over you.

Keep a written journal for one bad habit you want to change. For instance, if you are trying to quit smoking, what triggers you to smoke? Do you smoke at certain times of the day? Are there certain people you smoke around? Do you smoke more often after a tense episode at work or home? Finding out "when" and "why" gives you more power to change.

Change is seen as threatening because it intrudes into our comfort zone. Change in and of itself is not bad, just different.

When changing a habit, don't expect perfection. If you slip, forgive yourself and keep trying. You haven't failed until you've failed to try.

"If you are heading in the wrong direction, God allows U-turns."
—*From a bumper sticker*

Conscious of Consequences

Many years ago Harry Emerson Fosdick told the story of a man who got on a bus with the intention and desire of going to Detroit. When he arrived at the end of a long, tiring journey, he found he was not in Detroit, but was in Kansas City. At first, he refused to believe it. When he asked for Woodward Avenue and was told there was no Woodward Avenue, he was indignant. It was quite some time before this man could face the fact that in spite of his good intentions and earnest desires, he was not in Detroit at all, but was indeed in Kansas City. You see he had made one small mistake. He had taken the wrong bus.

Often there are similar situations in our own lives. We all want the good things life has to offer: success, a fine home, a loving family, competence in our work, the respect of friends, an honorable name, a healthy body, and a long life. Yet, nothing is more common than unfilled desires and unrealized good intentions. We may have the most worthwhile goals and the finest plans, and we may be thinking about a wonderful destination. But, if we take the wrong bus, we may very well end up in a place where we don't want to be. No matter how good our intentions are, they don't help much if we take a road that leads to somewhere else.

Traveling along the road of life should be like a safe journey taken in an automobile. When traveling in a car, we have to stop often to fill our vehicle with fuel, check the tires, wash the windows, and perhaps add oil or other additives that our car may require. We also need to stop to refresh and refuel ourselves. Accidents can happen if we become too tired and are not as alert as we need to be. What we do along the way will many times reflect what the end of the journey will be like. Our desires and good intentions will not matter if we haven't taken the necessary steps to arrive in safety.

So it is with our everyday journey of life. We need to check ourselves to see if we are on the right road, taking the necessary precautions, to arrive safely at the end of a long, happy, fulfilling, healthy life. Ponder the following questions:

- Am I taking care of myself?
- Am I getting sufficient sleep?
- Am I eating the right foods?
- Am I staying out of the sun?
- Am I getting adequate exercise?
- Am I being positive about life?
- Do I have faith in tomorrow?
- Am I taking control of my life, or am I just waiting for "things" to happen?

It is important to understand, that what we do today really matters. We get to make choices about what we do on a daily basis; but, we don't get to choose the consequences.

No one wants to get cancer, and yet people smoke a pack of cigarettes a day. No one wants to have a stroke or a heart attack, yet there are people who are 75 pounds overweight, eating like there's no tomorrow. There are those who want to look young and vital, and spend hours sunbathing until their skin is the texture of leather. There are those who desire energy and vitality who have indentations in their couches from sitting in front of the television set day after day after day.

If you want to live a longer, healthier, happier life, then do something about it! Golda Meir stated, "Nothing in life just happens. You have to have the stamina to meet the obstacles and overcome them."

I submit that there's a time in all our lives when we need to stop, regroup, and examine the road we are traveling on. Are we on the right "bus?" Are we traveling safely? Are our good intentions in sync with our actions? Or, do we need to get off at the next stop? Do we need to make a U-turn and head in a new direction?

I assure you that the road to a happy, healthy, fulfilling life is out there. There is no rush hour, and it is rarely congested. My wish is that each of us will have the strength to put our good intentions and actions on the right road that will take us to our chosen destination. Then years from now, when we look back at the life we've lived and the choices we've made, we'll be exactly where we wanted to be.

Forever Facts:

Check the signs on your path of life. Are you traveling where you want to be?

Ask yourself if a few course corrections would improve your life.

Your behavior is your choice. The consequences resulting from your behavior are not.

*"The saddest thing in life is when the man you are
meets the man you might have become."*
—*Unknown*

Get Going with Goals

A far-sighted man determined that he was going to work hard, earn a significant sum of money, and then retire early and enjoy life. When he did retire, he was miserable. It wasn't that he missed the every day rat race or the congested commute. It wasn't that he missed the thrust and parry of business negotiations. What he missed was the sense of purpose. Now that he was retired, he was floundering. He was like a rudderless boat aimlessly floating on the current here and there, without really going anywhere. He had set goals for himself that he had accomplished, and now he had nothing to work for. The mistake this man had made was not setting new goals and not reframing his sense of purpose.

We can all have a purposeful existence by setting goals in our life. Goals are specific objectives, attained through concrete action. "If you can't measure it, rate it or describe it, it is probably not a goal," said Michael LeBoeuf, a New Orleans business consultant.

There are many people whose lives have benefited from goal setting. Read their stories below and profit from their advice.

- **Define Your Objective**
  Dave Thomas, the late owner and memorable advertiser for the Wendy's restaurant chain, wanted to own

his own restaurant from the time he was eight years old. Orphaned at birth, Thomas never had a stable home life. He wanted to own a restaurant because that way, he said, "I'd never be hungry."

Thomas clung to his goal. When he was 12, he got a job as a counterman in a diner. Later, he worked his way up from busboy to a restaurant manager. Thomas turned around four failing fried-chicken restaurants and became an executive with a national chain.

Finally, after putting together the necessary capital, he eventually opened his own place in Columbus, Ohio, and named it after his daughter Wendy. Today there are more than 3,800 Wendy restaurants.

Thomas advised, "I didn't set my sights on owning 1,000 restaurants or even ten. I just concentrated on making one profitable, then another, one step at a time."

We need to know what we want to achieve, and then go forward with concrete steps to accomplish it.

- **Put It on Paper**

  Once you've defined your goal, write it down. High achievers trace their accomplishments to the time they committed their goals to paper. Write it down and carry it with you wherever you go. Take it out of your pocket, look at it, and think about it. As you do, evaluate it and see how you are progressing. A great religious leader, speaking to a group of youth about setting goals in their lives, stated, "A goal is only a wish unless it is written down."

- **Map Out Your Strategy**

  Curtis Carlson, founder of the Gold Bond Stamp Company in Minneapolis, has some great ideas on mapping out your strategy for accomplishing a goal. He says, "Breaking a goal down into bite-size pieces makes achieving it seem less intimidating." Backward planning, which consists of setting an objective and then retracing the steps needed to achieve it, is a successful technique for many.

- **Set a Deadline**

  "A goal is a dream with a deadline," says motivational speaker, Zig Zigler. Deadlines provide a time frame for action and spur you on in pursuit of your dreams. When you reach the deadline you've set for a goal, review your goal and what you've done to achieve it. If you haven't attained your goal, maybe changes need to be made. Annotate the changes, set a new deadline, and then go forward.

- **Commit Yourself**

  Success is something we create for ourselves. Some may have a structured routine and others a "vision." Writing down a goal is not enough, nor is knowing what steps to take or setting a deadline. What brings about success is implementing the steps needed to accomplish your goal. Tom Landry, a legendary coach of the Dallas Cowboys football team, believed: "Setting a goal is not the [only] thing. It is deciding how you will go about achieving it and staying with that plan."

- **Don't Fear Failure**

  Think of goal setting as starting out on a long journey to somewhere you have never been before. There may be detours, setbacks or obstacles along the way, but that doesn't mean the destination won't be reached. Thomas Edison put the fear of failure into perspective when he said; "I haven't failed. I've found 10,000 ways that don't work."

- **Never Give Up**

  Believe in yourself! That belief can act as an analgesic when setbacks come. Envision yourself being successful. Encourage yourself on the pathway to success. "You can't lose until you quit trying," Benjamin Franklin assured.

  Winston Churchill expressed Franklin's sentiment a little differently but every bit as effectively when he spoke at a school in England. He probably gave the shortest talk in history; but he also gave one of the most profound and meaningful. Churchill approached the podium, looked around at the students, and then succinctly stated, "Never give up. Never give up. Never, never, never give up." The Prime Minister then bid the students and faculty farewell and left the room. This eleven-word speech, although brief, has gone down in the annals of history. Its message is as meaningful today as on the day it was delivered.

A lot of times, we think of goals as only having meaning for and being beneficial to those on the threshold of life. From my childhood, I learned and still believe that everyone, no matter what his or her age, benefits from working towards something. In fact, envisioning work that still needs to be done and goals that still need to be set is probably one of the more effective anti-aging applications in existence.

This is confirmed by the war-time experiences of Victor Frankl, an Austrian psychologist, who survived the death camps of Nazi Germany. As Frankl found within himself the capacity to rise above his humiliating circumstances, he became an observer as well as a participant in the experience. He watched others who shared in the ordeal and was intrigued with the question of what made it possible for some people to survive when most died.

Frankl looked at several factors: health, vitality, family structure, intelligence, and survival skills. Finally, he concluded that none of these factors was primarily responsible. The single most significant factor, Frankl realized, was a sense of future vision. Those who managed to survive had the compelling conviction that they still had a mission to perform, some important work left to do.

Looking at our lives and finding things we still need to accomplish and work toward can, in effect, become the DNA of our lives. Seeing the need to set goals, work, and move forward can become the compelling impetus behind every decision we make.

Setting goals not only gives us a sense of purpose, helps us find success, and increases our life span, but it also refines our personalities. Ghandi, who came from a background of timidity, scarcity, fear, jealousy, and insecurity, basically didn't even want to be with people. He preferred being left alone. He didn't like working as a lawyer until he gradually began to find some satisfaction in helping both sides win. As he began to see the injustices of the Indian people, however, a vision was born in his mind and heart. Out of that vision came the goal of helping the Indian people transform themselves. Ghandi was driven to help his people develop a sense of self-worth and to stop seeing themselves as inferior to their British overlords.

As Ghandi focused on his goal, his personality weaknesses were essentially eclipsed. Vision and purpose created personality growth and development. He wanted not only to love people, but also to serve and be with people. As a result, he eventually brought England to its knees and freed three hundred million people. Ghandi remarked, "I claim to be no more than an average man with below average capabilities. I have not the shadow of a doubt that any man or woman can achieve what I have if he or she would put forth the same effort and cultivate the same hope and faith."

Or, in other words, anyone can accomplish anything great if they set a goal and are willing to work to achieve it. And the feeling that comes from successful accomplishment is surely the equivalent of a sip at the Fountain of Youth. As Samuel Johnson said, "Life affords no higher pleasure than that of surmounting difficulties, passing from one step of success to another, forming new wishes and seeing them gratified." Whatever your age, if you utilize the goal-setting strategies outlined above, you can move ever onward and upward in life.

Forever Facts:

You haven't been defeated until you quit trying.

No matter what your age, station, or situation in life, following goal-setting strategies can help your life improve.

To accomplish a goal, you need to set small, do-able steps, while never losing sight of the ultimate objective.

Even an elephant can be eaten, one bite at a time.

Part Three

"Attitudes of Aging"

I believe certain attitudes and mindsets regarding aging are detrimental to us. I would like to suggest specific areas where attitude adjustments toward the aging process would reap great benefits.

*"The older I grow the more I distrust the familiar doctrine
that age brings wisdom."*
—H. C. Mencken

Your Genes Won't Kill You

In the "Four Basic Theories of Aging" chapter, I discuss genetic research and how it can affect the aging process. However, I realize that there are those who believe they have already figured out the role of genetics in aging. They think it's deadly. There are those who are well-informed about family deaths and illnesses, and see themselves fatalistically getting each and every one. These are the individuals who make such comments as, "By the time anyone in my family reaches 40 they start going downhill," or "I'm just like my father. He died at 72, so I worry I won't be around to take care of my wife."

Too often, many of us, when reaching a certain age, adopt a mindset which starts with thinking of our parents' lives: how long they lived, their cause of death, etc. We immediately start calculating our life span to coincide with that of our parents, which can be misleading and even detrimental.

With such feelings already inherent in us, it is a certainty that with every pain thereafter, we will immediately see the scenario of "must haves." For instance, if I am feeling a pain in my knee, I could start to think, "My father was crippled with arthritis. He started out with pains in his knees. I *must have* arthritis. It will get continually worse, and then one day I will end up in a wheelchair, dying before my 69th birthday just like Dad."

Well-ingrained in the mentality of "my genes are going to

be the death of me," we start enumerating other genetic "age" symptoms, such as thinning and graying hair, memory lapses, and sagging skin. Now certain that we have arthritis, we start protecting the sore knee. Getting stiff from protecting the knee, it now hurts to exercise, so the exercising stops. We are sitting more, gradually decreasing our activity. We get more and more stiff from just sitting and, consequently, it becomes more difficult to move around at all. Now the reality is not a happy one. At first, a cane is needed to improve mobility, then gradually a walker is required, and, finally, a wheelchair, where we await the grim reaper.

When we have the expectation of becoming crippled with age, that is exactly what happens. Every little pain and ache becomes a "must have" and, with our imagination allowed to run rampant, we become victims of self-fulfilling prophecy.

It is a cinch that we all have some predisposition to one thing or another. However, I can assure you that a predisposition is not a certainty. Just because our parents or grandparents lived to a certain age, that doesn't mean our life span is already predetermined to coincide with theirs.

Certainly there are scientists who believe that our life span is affected by what they call "programmed senescence," which is based on the belief that aging results from a genetic program. Others argue other aging factors are more dominant (see "Four Basic Theories of Aging" on page 15). Most scientists will agree that a variety of elements contribute to our aging process. But, while each idea can be analyzed, I remind you that nothing can be predicted precisely.

There are definitive examples of genetics NOT relating to life span. In one family, twin boys grew up together in the same surroundings, eating the same diet, getting similar exercise, etc. One brother died at 35, while the other lived to the age of 92. The brothers' longevity could not have been related to their parents, because their parents died a year apart in their late 60's.

Another example is a young woman, who, when approaching her fortieth birthday, was filled with dread that she would die of a brain tumor. Her mother had died at that age with a brain tumor, leaving behind a husband and eight children, with the youngest being only 18 months old. This woman was certain that she was genetically predisposed to share a similar fate. Her fortieth birthday came and went without so much as a headache. However, the stress from worry and fear over dying and leaving her husband and children probably contributed to future emotional problems that she is still battling.

Contrast the above with an example from an earlier generation, in the days when there was little treatment available for cancer. A young woman, recently married, took care of her 40-year-old mother until she died of breast cancer. This woman got breast cancer herself at the age of 60, then 12 years later Lymphoma. She went through radiation treatment for breast cancer and chemotherapy in her battle against Lymphoma. Both treatments were extremely hard on her body, but she is cancer-free and alive and well today. She will eagerly share her ideas for survival, which are especially pertinent to the anti-aging approach.

Her suggestions include eating a wide variety of fruits and vegetables and avoiding fat in the diet. She is quick to point out that it is also important to have a daily diet of cheerfulness. She is a firm believer that an optimistic attitude and a determination to overcome and succeed were not only significant aids in her overcoming cancer, but are also strong deterrents to her "getting old." Now at age 73, she is doing great and planning her 100th birthday. She firmly believes that "to live long, one must start young."

When considering the issue of longevity, instead of focusing on genetics and trying to fit ourselves into our parents' pattern, it would be infinitely more helpful to develop a healthy physical and emotional lifestyle and set a pattern of our own. As Dag Hammarskjold once said, "We are not permitted to choose the frame of our destiny. But what we put into it is ours."

I am a firm believer that instead of focusing on the "must haves" or "what ifs" of genetics, we need to focus on what *we* can do today. Elizabeth Barrett Browning said it best when she advised, "Light tomorrow with today."

Forever Facts:

Fear is ousted by fact. If you feel you have a predisposition toward an illness, do some research and talk to your doctor.

Genetics are no match for a positive mindset.

Don't borrow trouble.

Develop a healthy lifestyle that will allow you to graft a long, healthy branch on the family tree.

*"The three ages of man are youth, middle age,
and you're looking wonderful."*
—Red Skelton

Breaking Out of the Aging Trap

In the movie, *Rocky*, the title character, Rocky Balboa, is a broken-down, "never was" part-time boxer and part-time "too nice" collection agent for a local loan shark. He's never had much in the way of worldly goods or education. Rocky fits the stereotype of someone from a lower class neighborhood, who was born in a poor part of town and plans on dying there. When we first meet Rocky, his expectations for himself are closely aligned to the stereotypical prospects of someone born in his class. He views himself as basically a "bum" and anticipates remaining that way.

Now *Rocky* is a fictitious story, and, you might dismiss the idea of someone placing limitations on himself because of stereotypical thinking. However, people every day allow themselves to be influenced by "what is expected of them." This, unfortunately, it is all too real and all too common.

This has particular application regarding those who are middle age and older. Individuals in this age range may find themselves slipping into the "Aging Trap," due to stereotypes about getting older.

Go into any party store, and you will find a section dedicated to "over the hill" birthday festivities. There are black balloons to mark the occasion, birthday cards with snide quips about aging, and funeral paraphernalia to make sure that every birthday you celebrate past the age of 40 makes you feel really, *really* old.

139

If the birthday celebration doesn't push you into a stereo-typical mindset regarding getting older, then a visit to your doctor will probably do the trick. It is sad—but true—that there are physicians out there (usually under the age of 30, fresh from medical school) who will make such comments as, "Well at 'your age' (heavy emphasis on AGE), you have to expect a few aches and pains." Then your eye doctor will tell you to get ready to wear bi- or trifocals, "because that is a reality for someone who's as old as you are."

You don't have to be a plastic surgeon to realize that in our society today, the "young and beautiful" are revered. Ask a random group of people if they consider looks as a factor in their determinations about the mental spryness of an older person. They may answer that youth and physical attractive-ness are not considerations; however, psychological experiments show just the opposite. Attractive, younger people are often perceived as mentally sharper than older, less attrac-tive people.

Youth is also valued by corporate America. Businesses today seem to value younger, inexperienced, cheaper employees over those with tenure, benefits, and higher salaries. The suggested and mandatory retirement programs are structured to clear out the older worker to make the way for the graduates, fresh from college.

There are also those old age jokes and quips delivered by twenty-something comedians that can be deflating to the spirit. And then, by the time you explain to your grandson that no, you *weren't* alive when George Washington was President, you're feeling pretty ancient.

The danger with the "Aging Trap" mindset is that you can get caught in it and come to believe the aging stereotypes. You see the aches and pains, the frailty, the diminished mental capacity, the physical slowdown, etc. as being inevitable, which is far from the truth. As a consequence, as you age, you stop doing the things you enjoy that have kept you young and active. You then settle down to the business of aging, which, in effect, hastens the aging process. Evidence has shown that those who are positive about aging and keep themselves busy live a much longer, healthier life.

In an assisted living facility, the social director continually told the older residents how wise they were and how much she enjoyed being with them. She would ask their advice about her children and other issues in her life. From the efforts of this social director to make the tenants feel needed, appreciated, and valued, they blossomed. They became more positive in their outlook, much happier about their lives, and reduced their complaining about everything.

Since aging is something we all hope to experience, it behooves us to learn all we can about the aging process. Many of our preconceived notions about aging diminish with knowledge and understanding.

A beautiful essay on aging, written by M.E.K. Fisher, when she was in her seventies, gives us a charming glimpse of life as we get older. Ms. Fisher wrote:

> Parts of the aging process are scary, of course, but the more we know about them, the less they need to be. That is why I wish we were more deliberately taught, in early years, to prepare for that condition. It would leave a lot of us freed to enjoy the obvious rewards of being old, when the sound of a child's laugh, or the catch of sunlight on a flower petal is as poignant as ever was a girl's voice to an adolescent boy's ear, or the tap of a golf ball into its cup to a balding banker's. ... We are unprepared for the years that may come as our last ones. Plainly, I think this clumsy modern pattern is a wrong

one, an ignorant one, and I regret and wish that I could
do more to change it.

Too often, our ideas about aging are inaccurate based on
hurtful and destructive stereotypes, which need to be recognized for what they are. We need to rid ourselves of the
paradigm that defines people by age. It's important to value the
seasoned, mature individuals in our society, recognizing they
can bless our lives with a wealth of information and knowledge
from having experienced and survived the goodness and the
harshness of life. And, as we age, we need to appreciate those
same qualities and aspects about ourselves.

David Mahoney and Richard Restak, M.D. believe that
when we think of preparing for aging, we normally focus on
taking care of financial needs. Of course, it's important to start
saving and investing early in our careers, so, at retirement age,
the needed funds will be available. However, Mahoney and
Restak point out that there are some who work to retire as soon
as possible, never planning how their time will be spent after
they quit working. Oftentimes, health problems arise from a
lack of exercise, and discouragement occurs from a lack of
things to do.

Americans are starting to recognize the need to prepare for
aging mentally, emotionally, and physically. Disability rates in
Americans older than 65 dropped 15 percent between 1982 and
1994, according to scientists in the Duke University Center for
Demographic Studies.

Smarter, healthier living is responsible for this improvement, according to Kenneth G. Manton, the professor who
oversaw the Duke study. These results don't factor in the recent
medical advances in aging, which would probably improve the
numbers even more.

We can be healthier, live longer, and be more positive about aging. Sister Mary Gemma Brunke writes beautifully about the upside of aging:

> *It is the old apple trees that are decked with the loveliest blossoms.*
>
> *It is the ancient redwoods that rise to majestic heights.*
>
> *It is the old violins that produce the richest tones.*
>
> *It is the aged wine that tastes the sweetest.*
>
> *It is ancient coins, stamps and furniture that people seek.*
>
> *It is the old friends that are loved the best.*

Thank God for the blessings of age and the wisdom, patience and maturity that go with it. Old is wonderful!

As the movie *Rocky* progresses, Rocky Balboa gets a chance to go up against the champ. His stereotypical thinking changes and his hope increases. He starts working and challenging himself. From this point on in the movie, we see Rocky training and are able to monitor his improvement through his increased speed and stamina. One of the most inspirational scenes in the movie is when Rocky, who has formerly stumbled up the front stairs of a large building in downtown Philadelphia, is finally able to run to the top of the steps. In this affecting moment of triumph, he raises his arms high above his head in victory. At the close of the movie, Rocky ends up losing to the champ, but that really doesn't matter; because Rocky has burst the bands of stereotypical thinking and has triumphed over himself.

It is critical that each of us rids ourselves of stereotypical thinking in regards to aging. We need to determine to be the best we can be at any age, and work to achieve our own victory over self. Remember: "Beautiful people are acts of nature, but beautiful, *old* people are works of art."

Forever Facts:

The most important planning for old age is NOT financial.

Victory over self is the greatest achievement of all.

Instead of reminding yourself that you're getting older, remind yourself of how far you've come in terms of wisdom, maturity, knowledge, insight, understanding, development of talents, etc.

A smarter, healthier lifestyle leads to a longer, healthier, life.

"They can conquer who believe they can."
— *Virgil*

How to Look in the Mirror and Like What You See

When you look in the mirror who and what do you see? Do you see this confident person who knows where they are going, and who has plans made and goals set to arrive at his or her desired location?

There is a long-time, ongoing debate regarding which has the most influence in the making of "you," environment or heredity. Regardless of which side of the argument you align yourself with, there is a certainty that "you are an original and not a paint by number."

I was blest to have a wonderful, supportive family while growing up. However, if you didn't, that does not earmark you to be a failure in the future! I encourage everyone who reads this book to remember you have the power to become anything you choose to be. Certain situations in life may require a little more effort to overcome than others. Let me point out, however, that you can and will be successful if you are willing to do your best and spend the time needed to work toward the goals you have chosen.

Whenever we examine heredity, we need to factor in our divine heritage that enables us to rise above anything. Many years ago a very successful woman, successful in the things of life that really count, had a formula she lived by and handed down to her children. Her formula was "Me + God = Enough."

She said that "Me" comes first in the formula because we first have to be willing to do our part. If we do all we can do, and then exercise faith, "God" will help us create a successful equation, one that will be "Enough" for us to accomplish anything we choose to strive for. This woman also realized and wanted her children to understand, just as my Mother did, that everyone has a cheering section available to them, "a Heavenly Father, who is always there."

Even if we have some negatives on our family tree, we can take advantage of our environment. Do you associate with confident people who seem to know where they are going? Are they people of integrity and high moral character? If so, learn from them. Just be sure you don't allow your self-image to be dictated by the opinions of others.

There is a story told about an Indian brave who found an eagle's egg and put it into the nest of a prairie chicken. The eaglet hatched with the brood of chicks and grew up with them. All his life, the changeling eagle, thinking he was a prairie chicken, did what the prairie chickens did. He scratched in the dirt for seeds and insects to eat. He clucked and cackled, and he flew as prairie chickens are supposed to fly in a brief thrashing of wings and flurry of feathers no more than a few feet off the ground. Years passed, and the changeling eagle grew very old. One day, he saw a magnificent bird far above him in the cloudless sky. Hanging with graceful majesty on the powerful wind currents, it soared with scarcely a beat of its strong wings. "What a beautiful bird!" said the changeling eagle to his neighbor. "What is it?"

"That's an eagle, chief of all birds," his neighbor clucked. "But don't give it a second thought. You could never be like him."

So the changeling eagle never did give it another thought. And it died thinking it was a prairie chicken. How sad when we allow others to determine what we become.

I want us to realize that a good self-image is really a matter of choice. We do not have to accept or believe what someone else says. Whether someone gives you a compliment or is rudely critical about you, it is your choice to accept or reject the comment.

When asked what the three most important words in the world are, most people would say, "I Love You." However, the three most important words in the world to help you become the best you can be are "**UP UNTIL NOW.**" Up until now . . . I was shy . . . or up until now I had no self-confidence, but that was yesterday. Now is today and NOW I will take control of my life, knowing I can accomplish anything I desire to do. I have the power within me to become anything I want to be. As the caption on a well-known poster says, "I'm somebody special 'cause God don't make no junk."

Although you may not be able to alter some of the situations in your life, you can certainly change the way you react to any event, regardless of its magnitude. Whatever labels we have worn in the past; we don't need to wear them in the future. As we change and grow, we can toss away those tags that no longer fit us. The following incident illustrates this point:

> For someone who tries so hard to be organized, I am often running to keep up. This morning was no different. Because of some unexpected interruptions, I was running late. I was due to attend a planning meeting for an upcoming luncheon to raise money for a local charity. Just as I slammed my car door, preparatory to taking off for the meeting, I realized I didn't have the crowd-pleasing recipe I promised to bring. I had found the recipe on the Internet, tried it, and knew it

would be perfect for the luncheon. Right at that moment I had no idea where I had put the recipe. I decided it would be faster to log onto my favorite food website again, rather than taking time to search the house. Watching the hands of the clock ticking by, I tried to log on to the website, when, to my frustration, I found I couldn't get on. The website was obviously under maintenance because instead of the site coming up, the words "UNDER CONSTRUCTION" flashed on my screen in big bold letters. Since I was now out of time, I rushed back to my car, hoping I would remember enough of the recipe to give the planning committee the idea. As I drove the 26 miles to the meeting, my mind kept flashing back to those two words in big bold letters "UNDER CONSTRUCTION." I realized I've been "under construction" all my life. I have always been working on a self-improvement program, and I will probably never be fully completed in my lifetime. But oh, what fun when I'm finally finished. I'll be like good wine, aged to perfection.

A number of years ago the General Electric Corporation appropriated a million dollars and allotted four years of time to research the importance of the human element in business success. The company had already spent large sums of money and a year of time in improving its manufactured products. Now it decided that more attention should be given to the improvement of the people who made, sold, and used the products. After several years of scientists working steadily, they determined that most human development comes from within the person himself.

I'd like to point out that some people have no direction in

life. They seem to wander around aimlessly, waiting for life successes to come their way. Juvenile authorities tell us that young teens get involved in drugs, alcohol, and other crimes because they have no direction. They have no self-respect, because they have no purpose. The same is true for adults. Those who wander aimlessly through life without purpose or a sense of self get trapped in feelings of inadequacy, enlarging their faults. We need to recognize that every person is born with or has developed different strengths and abilities.

This point is clearly made in the following story about the scientist, Dr. Henry Eyring. Dr. Eyring told of walking down a country road near Princeton University with the world-famous scientist, Albert Einstein. As they passed a field of hardy green plants, Dr. Eyring asked Einstein what the plants were. Einstein had lived in this area for some time. Dr. Eyring was new to the area, so he did not recognize the plants. Einstein had no idea what they were. Dr. Eyring, who had been raised on a farm, said he thought they were some kind of bean. After walking further, they came upon a man, sitting in a wheelbarrow. Dr Eyring asked his question of this man. The man replied, "'Oh, them! Them's soybeans." Einstein, who understood laws of the universe that even few scientists could comprehend, did not know a simple fact that the poor, uneducated man considered common knowledge. The poorest person may have some skill or knowledge that the wisest person does not have. Every one of us has limitations as well as strengths.

Try the following suggestions for improving your self-esteem:

Take Charge of Your Life

It has been said, "Life will give you whatever you are willing to accept." If you want to accept mediocrity or unhappiness or financial problems, that is exactly what life will let you have. If you want more, you can have that too, but you have to take charge of your life.

In his book, *Be Master of Yourself*, Robert L. Backman counsels:

> Achievement comes to those who push beyond their limitations, whatever they many be—those who work when they don't feel like it, those who believe when everything around them is faltering, those who hang on when hanging on seems almost too much. There is a great thrill in overcoming ourselves. It is far more difficult to master ourselves than to be master of a city —harder to discipline our weaknesses than to give in to them. It means to give up what we want this minute for what we want in the long run. It means to delay gratification when something sweet may be right at hand.

Realize That You Can Change

It makes no difference who you are or how old you may be. You can change directions and make your life better. Dream a little. If your dreams from years ago are no longer realistic, then replace them with something you can do right now. It's never too late to change, grow, and accomplish.

One young woman loved tennis and spent all her spare time in college enjoying the sport. When she married, she moved away from where tennis was easily accessible. Years went by. She felt the need for some exercise, and remembered the fun she had had with tennis. However, over the years, her vision had worsened, and it was harder to see the tennis ball coming over the net. Rather than giving up, however, this woman remembered she had also loved tap dancing. She went into a dance store and bought a pair of tap shoes with jingle taps. When she was alone, she would turn up the stereo, go into her garage, and tap up a storm. She found this impromptu, creative dancing not only refreshing and enjoyable, but wonderful exercise as well. One day this woman was enjoying herself so much she did not hear her husband come home from work. He heard the music and investigated. He was stunned. He gave his wife a hug and said, "You are great! Why didn't you tell me?"

Act as If

Jean is no beauty, but when she enters a room heads turn. What's her secret? Confidence. "I feel good about myself, and that carries over to how people feel about me," she says. If you walk with eyes alert, head up and shoulders back, and recognize people with a friendly smile, regardless of how insecure you feel, no one will ever know. Soon it will not be an act, it will be real.

Use Attitude Uplifts

Associate yourself with uplifting material. The refrigerator is the perfect background for an attitude uplift such as: "Happiness is self-inflicted." Don't stop with the kitchen. Post attitude uplift notes all over the house.

Associate yourself with positive people. It is hard to feel like a million bucks if someone is cutting you down. Cultivate relationships with people who value you and support you. Avoid those who are critical of others.

Count Your Successes

Compliment yourself. Value yourself. Don't wait for the roar of the crowd. Others are often too absorbed to give you the encouragement you deserve.

One woman was feeling under-appreciated and overworked. Leaving a store, she noticed an "Employee of the Week" certificate, honoring one of the store's employees. She went home, sat at her computer, and designed her very own "Employee of the Week" certificate, enumerating her contributions to her home and family. She posted it on the refrigerator, so that her husband could share in her honor. Her husband, when he noticed the certificate, rolled his eyes and shook his head. However, he still got the point. He started being more complimentary and acknowledging his wife's contributions.

You don't have to wait for others to make you feel good about you. Clap for yourself, and pat yourself on the back.

Self-Enlightenment

Many fill their life with so much "stuff" that there is no time or room left to become acquainted with themselves. It is important to take time for meditation, reflection, and self-evaluation. The more we come to know and value ourselves, the happier we are.

Learn As Long As You Live

There are a lot of people who, when they reach a certain age, believe they are too old to learn or think. This philosophy falls into the "you can't teach an old dog new tricks" pattern. When a new concept comes into their sphere of learning, some older individuals will balk and ask, "What good will this do me at my age?" Too many people narrow their scope more and more as they get older, instead of broadening it. It's important to keep learning and to develop the ability to always see the world with a fresh perspective.

To develop a positive feeling about ourselves, I submit there are six things to avoid that are detrimental to our self-image.

1. **Unrealistic Expectations**: Often we have focused in our minds the ideal way we should be in order to find success as a parent, friend, mother/father, wife/husband etc. When

we fall the least bit short, we feel we have failed. Then thoughts such as "I am not good, I am not capable," or "I will never make it" become a part of us. None of us are associating with perfect people today, so why, when we look in the mirror, do we expect that person to be perfect?

2. **Needless Guilt:** Guilt in and of itself can serve as a motivator. Looking into the past and wishing we had never made a certain mistake, however, is fruitless. When we look at the past, we need to learn from it. Guilt that prompts productive change is good. Guilt that anchors us in self-criticism is destructive.

3. **Needless Worry**: Guilt and worry destroy self-image. Guilt deals with the past, and worry deals with the future. Worry brings about anxiety or fear of future events. The confident person acts, while the unconfident one agonizes. Do you wonder how to overcome always anticipating the negative outcome? Consciously ask yourself "What is the worst that can happen?" Most likely it's something you can live with. Then ask yourself "What's the best possible outcome?" If you have to dwell on the answer to one of those two questions, dwell on the positive one.

4. **Comparisons**: If you want to be rid of never feeling inferior, then give up comparisons. You can't compare yourself to someone else because no two people are the same. A comparison is always inequitable because you see yourself at your worst, while viewing others at their best. The only person you should be competing against is you. Analyze what you did today, and then improve tomorrow.

5. **Seeking Immediate Perfection**: We want to lose 30 pounds yesterday. We pray to the Lord for patience, and ask for it tomorrow. Improvement and change are an ongoing process, not a destination.

6. Confusing Self-Worth with Behavior: Your self worth can never be eliminated. It is there just because YOU exist. To increase your own feelings of your self-worth, you must determine what is important to you and then set goals to achieve it. With each goal you accomplish, you will feel better about you.

I cannot emphasize enough the value and sanctity of life. It's important for each of us to remember that as far as life goes, there is only one to a customer. We need to start today to change what is holding us back from being the person we can be.

Someone has said, "We tend to act consistent with the way we see ourselves." This statement speaks to the extreme importance of recognizing our own true worth. In a religious magazine some years ago there was a thought-provoking quote that summarizes what we should feel when we look in the mirror: "Ponder the magnificence of what you see when you look in the mirror. Ignore the freckles, the unruly hair, or the blemishes, and look beyond to see the real you—not a paint by number but a true masterpiece. Believe, in yourself and live each day, striving to be all you are capable of becoming."

Forever Facts:

It has been estimated by psychologists that every time you make a negative, critical comment to someone, you have to make ten positive comments to balance out the effect. Remember that the next time you criticize yourself.

Environmental factors cannot conquer the power of personality.

Most of the limitations place on an individual are self-imposed.

*"A pessimist is one who feels bad when he feels good for
fear he'll feel worse when he feels better."*
—*Anonymous*

Don't Turn to the Obituary Page First

Have you ever wondered about those who, when they reach
a certain age, pick up a newspaper and immediately turn to the
obituary section? They don't even glance at the headlines. They
are oblivious to the news on the front page. Instead, they are
reviewing the names listed, mentally tabulating who is still
around and who has passed on. Now, there is certainly nothing
wrong with showing an interest in others; and, sometimes, the
obituary page contains poignant, memorable details about the
lives of those who are no longer with us that can teach some
valuable life lessons.

However, there is a lot wrong if the person turning to the
obituary page is focusing on death, feeling their age, and
mentally seeing their name soon to be listed among the
deceased. There is a lot wrong with that kind of negative,
pessimistic thinking.

We could learn a valuable lesson from a sign posted on a
mall directory. A young student walked into a mall he had
never been to before. In a hurry, he immediately walked over to
the mall directory to find the location of the store that would be
likely to have what he needed. As he looked at the directory, he
noticed a sign taped on it that said, "You are here—this is where
you are currently standing—are you going to stroll through life
or are you going to go through it with *enthusiasm*?" Going
through life with enthusiasm is something I feel very strongly

about and believe we should each ask ourselves that same question.

Like everything else in life we have a choice about our mental attitude. It is our choice to be either optimistic or pessimistic. No one can force us to have one mindset or the other. However, the optimistic person, fired with enthusiasm, finds humor in life and is better able to rise above life's irritations and setbacks much better than the pessimist can.

A good example of optimism is found in the following true story of two friends. These two friends from childhood had always teased and tried to outdo each other with pranks. They grew to manhood, married, and went their separate ways. One became a builder and the other a mortician. Tom, the builder, could never seem to get the best of Bob, the mortician, no matter how hard he tried.

After marriage, Tom and his family moved to Teton Valley in Idaho, and, several years later, Bob moved his family to the same area to open a mortuary. The friendship continued, as well as the pranks with Bob always getting the best of Tom.

Both of these men loved horses, and Bob was constantly helping himself to Tom's bridles, saddles etc. without asking. This was irritating to Tom, and he was determined to put a stop to it. He had already changed the locks on his horse barn, but that hadn't even slowed Bob down.

As Christmas approached, Tom decided on a plan that he was sure, for once, would get the best of Bob. This plan had the added advantage of putting a stop to Bob's taking his riding equipment.

Tom took a box into his wife, Peggy, asking her to wrap it for him to deliver to Bob on Christmas Eve. She did a beautiful wrapping job, using colorful, seasonal paper and adorning the top with a large bow. Tom and Peggy stopped by to wish Bob and Tonya a wonderful Christmas, and Tom placed his gift for

Bob under the tree. As they drove away, Peggy, well aware of the pranks the two had pulled on each other over the years, began questioning her husband about the package. She was concerned that Tom was doing something that would jeopardize the friendship they both cherished with Bob and Tonya.

"For the first time in my life I am going to get the best of Bob," Tom told his wife. "I can hardly wait until morning when Bob opens my gift." At this point, Peggy was almost afraid to find out *what* her husband had given his friend.

Tom didn't have long to wait. Rather than his phone ringing Christmas morning, there was a knock on Tom's door. When Tom answered the door, he found his buddy Bob standing there with the biggest smile he had ever seen. Bob, the true optimist, said "Hey good buddy, what a friend you are! That was really clever. When I opened that box of manure, I just knew you were going to give me that horse of yours I've wanted forever. You are some friend!" The look on Tom's face spoke volumes. Bob exuded such optimism! And you guessed it! Bob enjoyed the horse for years.

Optimism creates joy at any age, and adds peace to every one of life's phases. As an optimistic person ages, he looks forward to the future with excitement for each and every turn of the road, even though he knows there will be bumps and detours along the way. His optimistic attitude helps him face and overcome difficult times.

If you think optimistically, you will act optimistically. An Irish proverb reveals that "a man becomes the song he sings," or, in other words, "fake it, till you make it." We need to remember that we can induce feelings in ourselves by acting like the feelings already exist. This isn't hypocrisy. This is another way to assist us in dwelling on the good rather than the negative.

It is extremely important that we develop a good, optimistic attitude towards life and the world. I am a firm believer that we need to set a positive example for the generations coming after us. There is nothing more common today than a cynical, pessimistic attitude. You only have to turn on the television set and watch five minutes of news to perceive that.

In a recent survey taken in a lockup facility for troubled youth, teens were interviewed and asked why they didn't smile. One youth answered, "What's there to smile about?" Pessimism exuded from him. In response to the question, "Who is your hero?" the answer was "no one."

What about each one of us? Do we have a hero? Are we up to being a hero for someone else? We can be a hero for future generations by facing life and it's problems with an unquench-able, optimistic attitude. We can show others, in the words of Ella Wheeler, that "there is nothing we cannot live down, rise above, and overcome."

I suggest the time is now to begin improving ourselves, our attitude, and our outlook on life. We need to go forward with a positive, optimistic outlook, and we need to let it show. We may be just the instrument to make a tremendous change, not only in ourselves, but also in our children, grandchildren, friends, and the stranger we smile at in the grocery store.

A young woman, who had accompanied her mother to a grocery store, watched as her mother's groceries were being checked out. This young woman became more infuriated by the minute at the rude way the clerk was speaking to her mother. When they got into the car, the daughter, who was very protec-tive of her mother, turned and said, "Mom, you don't even know when people are rude to you. That man back there was extremely rude, and you smiled and thanked him."

The mother just smiled and said, "Oh, I knew he was being rude, but I don't feel I need to retaliate in kind. I'm not willing to give him control over my life and me. In fact, I'm kind of sorry for him. He must be terribly sad to feel that he has to strike out at others."

There is a story told of a wise, old man who lived in Sicily at the time of Cicero. Because of his vast wisdom, people would come from miles around to converse with and gain advice from him. But, there was a group of rebellious youth in the city that wanted to prove the old man a fool. The leader of the group came up with a plan. He decided to capture a bird in his hands and take it to the old man. He would ask if the bird was dead or alive.

If the old man said it was alive, he would tighten his hands, crushing the life from the bird. If the man said it was dead, he would open his hands allowing the bird to fly away. Either way, the man would be proven a fool. So the boys made their way to the center of the city where the wise, old man was preaching. The leader of the group called out, "Old man, what do I have in my hands?" And the old man answered, "A bird, my son." "And, is it dead or is it alive?" sneered the leader. There was a pause, and then the man wisely answered, "It is up to you, my son. It is as you wish it."

We need to realize that in the final analysis, optimism or pessimism is our choice. We can choose to have a positive, happy outlook on life that brings joy to us and those around us. Or, we can choose to be negative and miserable and spread that misery to all with whom we come in contact. It's up to us. Our attitude will be as we wish it to be.

So, my question for each of us,
"What's it going to be—optimism or pessimism?
You choose!"

Forever Facts:
    Optimistic people live longer.
    Optimistic people are happier.
    Optimistic people are statistically more successful in overcoming and avoiding illness.

*"An archaeologist is the best husband any woman can have:
the older she gets, the more interested he is in her."*
—Agatha Christie

Lighten Up

In 1964, a crippling disease of the connective tissues struck Norman Cousins. His spine and joints were so inflamed that just turning over in bed caused him pain. Still, he swore off analgesics and instead prescribed for himself massive doses of Vitamin C, along with "gobs of humor." Cousins remembers:

> I laughed my way through reruns of Allan Funt's *"Candid Camera"* and Marx Brothers' and Three Stooges' movies. I made the joyous discovery that ten minutes of genuine laughter had an anaesthetic effect and would give me at least two hours of pain-free sleep. When the painkilling effect of the laughter wore off, we would switch on the motion picture projector again and, not infrequently, it would lead to another pain-free interval.

"Laughter is good—it's like running or swimming or rowing," says William F. Fry, M.D., associate clinical professor of psychiatry at Stanford University. According to Dr. Fry's research, laughter increases the heart rate, works the muscles in your face and stomach, enhances circulation, and quickens breathing. A good laugh also ventilates the lungs, because you exhale more air than normal and breathe in fresh oxygen. When the laughter subsides, the body enters a relaxed state.

For a few seconds, blood pressure, breathing, and heart rate all fall below normal levels, and muscle tension disappears. And, research suggests the effect may be cumulative, like the benefits of exercise.

One of the most valuable health supplements I could prescribe would be mega doses of "mirth." Tests have shown that when humor is a part of daily life there is an increase of immunoglobulin A, which fights off upper respiratory infections, a decrease in the use of antidepressants, and a detoxification of the body. Laughter is our first line of defense against sickness brought on by unrelieved frustration and anger. Crying keeps us human, but laughing keeps us well.

Humor can also help us minimize errors. Experts say people make more mistakes and have more accidents when they're tense. By laughing at ourselves, we release some of the tension and reduce our risk of failure.

I agree with experts who say that people who can laugh at themselves are also more likely to make friends. Why? Because people who can laugh at themselves are seen by others as more human, warmer, more confident, and more accepting. "When you laugh at yourself, people assume that you're not going to judge them too harshly either," explains Joyce Anisman-Saltman, special education professor at Southern Connecticut State University in New Haven. "That puts people at ease, It gives them permission not to be perfect."

Birds can fly because they take themselves lightly. There are things in life that need our serious attention, such as work and responsibilities; but, the one thing we should never take seriously is ourselves. Laughing at oneself is one of life's noblest and most difficult acts. It takes courage and intelligence to recognize our own foolishness and deflate our own pretensions.

Some experts believe that humor and other positive feelings can free the mind from its usual patterns of logic, switching it into a more imaginative mode. When we are in this freer state, we are better able to approach problems creatively. Humor allows us to better utilize problem-solving capabilities.

According to polls, laughter is also prized in the workplace. "People with a sense of humor do better at their jobs than those who have little or no sense of humor," states Psychologist Barbara Mackoff, Ph.D. It is found that people with a sense of humor tend to be more creative, less rigid, and more willing to consider and embrace new ideas and methods. "What's more, the stress-defusing element of laughter can actually help you perform better on the job by boosting your energy and preventing burn-out," Mackoff adds. Research has also shown that humor can help you recover more quickly from mistakes.

Humor can even help establish your authority. "Women often feel that they won't be taken seriously if they are funny," says Mackoff, "but nothing could be further from the truth. Showing a sense of humor bespeaks credibility, confidence, and ease about you. It is the ultimate professional polish."

Laughter helps us feel better about ourselves. "When we laugh at our flaws and failures, we put them in perspective," says women's humor specialist, Regina Barreca, professor of English at the University of Connecticut. "I compare it to seeing a monster on a movie screen. It looks huge until the camera pulls back. You suddenly see that the monster is nothing but a hand puppet. Laughter works the same way," she says. "If you can laugh at a vexing situation, you cut it down to size."

I sincerely believe that laughter is also one of the best self-confidence builders there is. A few years ago, a couple was celebrating their Golden Wedding Anniversary. Their children planned and carried out a reception in their honor. As part of the festivities, the couple's children had put together a program about their parents. The program consisted of favorite music from the parents' era, incidents from their lives, memories of lessons learned and examples benefited from, and stories that had kept the couple's children and grandchildren laughing for years. One memory that was especially a hit was related by the couple's oldest granddaughter.

Standing before approximately 300 friends and relatives of her grandparents, the oldest granddaughter approached the microphone. She told of her grandmother taking her on a trip to Texas via airplane. On the way home, as her grandmother was walking down the airplane aisle after a quick visit to the restroom, growing chuckles and giggles attracted the grand-daughter's attention. Turning around in her seat to see where the laughter was coming from, she realized that all the people on the airplane were laughing as her grandmother walked down the aisle. As her grandmother sat down, she realized why the people were laughing. Her grandmother had tucked her dress and slip into the back of her panty hose.

As the granddaughter came to the end of her anecdote, the crowd in the reception hall burst into laughter. Most of the people attending the Golden Wedding reception viewed the grandmother as a dignified, "all together" type of lady. This story proved that she was also a *human* lady. Every person in the crowd could relate, in some degree or another, to an expe-rience when they had been less than their best, appearing even a little foolish.

A few years later, while shopping, the grandmother happened to meet one of the friends who had attended the Golden Wedding program. The two women visited, inquiring into the latest happenings of each other's lives. Before leaving, the friend confided, "Of all the things I have attended in my lifetime, I have never enjoyed anything as much as you and your husband's Golden Wedding Anniversary party. One of the things I will never forget is your granddaughter's story of your airplane bathroom visit. From your experience, I am learning to laugh at myself and to not take life so seriously. Thanks to you and your granddaughter, my self image has taken a growth spurt."

The following story sums up the overall benefit of a sense of humor:

It was only supposed to take a couple of hours for the mechanic to check my car over. However, the loud speaker summoned me to the service counter where I was told: "Mrs. Dexter, after checking the computer, we found there are 3 recalling notices rather than two. It will probably take about 4 _ hours to make the changes. We will be more than happy to take you anywhere you would like to go in the shuttle, or we can reschedule you for another time."

Since the garage was 24 miles from my home and since I was already there, I opted for the shuttle ride. The service manager told me that the shuttle had just arrived, and that the driver would be glad to take me anywhere I wanted to go. The shuttle driver, Hank, approached. He bent over, swinging his right arm in front of him in a half bow. "Your wish is my command, Ma'am!" he smilingly said. This brought a chuckle from those standing nearby. As I reached for the seat belt, Hank asked, "So, where would you like to go in our fair city?" His happy chatter was infectious.

"How about taking me to the library," I replied. "I need to do some research."

"Research? What kind?" Hank asked as he pulled into the library parking lot.

I explained I was working on a book, telling him

that I needed to verify my facts. "I never want to print anything without verification."

"Wow, that sounds really hard," Hank replied. "I'm not much of a reader. In fact, I don't like to read anything that doesn't make me laugh," he said.

As I prepared to get out of the shuttle, I turned to thank Hank and said, "Hank, I have the feeling you are a really happy person."

"Yes, ma'am, I really am," he answered. "Laughter sets everything all right with the world. There's too much sadness." Hank jumped out and hurried around to open my door. He took my bag and assisted me out of the van.

"Hank thanks for the ride and for your reminder, too. I'm going to take your advice and see what I can do to help set things 'all right' with the world."

I found myself smiling as I approached the information desk. I didn't think the library would have a book about 'setting everything all right with the world' so I just asked for directions to find a book on—you guessed it—the benefits of laughter.

Forever Facts:

It takes less muscles to smile than it does to frown.

Laughter has psychological, as well as physical benefits.

Crying makes us human, but laughing keeps us well.

Part Four

"Ageless Possibilities"

I believe that we need to focus on the ageless possibilities life has to offer. Making the most of life requires us to develop a philosophy that will govern our attitudes, actions, and choices. To truly value life, we must recognize it is a gift and treat it as such.

"Write your plans in pencil, in case you need to use an eraser."
— V. Richardson

Philosophy of Life

Through my life experiences, medical training, and personal philosophy, I have drafted a blueprint on how to conduct my life, which makes me feel healthy, happy, and productive. I trust each reader realizes that life is truly the most precious gift we have. I hope each of us will utilize that knowledge and search for the "forever factor," improving the quality of our lives.

Life is a precious gift, but it is not fair. Some of the things I have witnessed as a physician makes me realize that some are blessed with more worldly goods than others, some with more talents and abilities, some with a more positive outlook, etc. But, there is something that each and every one of us received as a free ticket along with this earthly experience. Each of us got the gift of free agency, the power of choice, to decide how we are going to live each day of our lives. We need to recognize the responsibility of life and take it seriously.

One of the things that my mother often reiterated to me was to "always remember God." We will value life more and understand it for the gift that it is if we recognize that there is a higher power, who is aware of each of us, who has granted us the privilege of life.

I know that we each have a responsibility to make the most of our own lives, but we were not left alone. To help in the actual realization of our divine destiny, Deity has implanted in every human soul a kind of "growth instinct," which Harry

Kemp calls *"The Upward Reach."* This inspired ambition for better things helps to make our lives more productive than they would otherwise be. Sterling W. Sill, explains in his book The Upward Reach, that "the chief instrument of every individual success is that eternal, forward, upward driving power within the seeker himself. The stimulation that we get from living at our best produces a great power within us. And, except for this internal striving, much of our ability would lie dormant forever."

I fervently believe that life is the greatest gift we can have. It behooves us to raise our standards, to reach higher in every phase of our lives to attain the greatest significance. It is by our own efforts that we grow—that we keep our growth instinct strong. To reach our destiny, a grounded character must underlie and stand behind every thought and act. It must dominate our work, our play, our worship, and our hopes. We must raise our sights, not settling for mediocrity, but making more effective demands upon ourselves. We must learn to take a more vigorous and effective action to get our personal life program in force.

We have within us all of the potentialities we need to accomplish something meaningful and worthwhile with our lives. We possess within ourselves those natural, inborn qualities of integrity, honor, compassion, and justice that can help us make the most of this gift of life. We need to ask ourselves the following questions: "What can I do with my life? What is my charge, my mission, my passion?" Then we need to develop our own talents and abilities to their utmost, using them to leave this life better than we found it and to find joy and peace in the process.

I would like to recommend these instructions for living a long, happy life:

"Whatsoever things are true,

Whatsoever things are honest,

Whatsoever things are just,

Whatsoever things are pure,

Whatsoever things are lovely,

Whatsoever things are of good report;

If there be any virtue;

And if there be any praise,

Think on these things."

Someone has said, "I like the approval of that important little night watchman of the soul called conscience." The conscience is a divine invention pointing us upward. We all like to win, and we are happy when we succeed. And, as my mother, Carmelita taught me, God is happy when we do, too.

Forever Facts:

Life is a gift!

Life has more meaning as we infuse more meaning into it.

Acceptance of mediocrity hastens aging.

Striving for excellence invigorates the spirit, mind, and body.

"Where there is love, there is life."
—*Mahatma Gandhi*

"Love is a Many-Splendored Thing"

Henry Drummond's literary masterpiece, *The Greatest Thing in the World*, responds to questions such as, What is the supreme good in the world? What is the noblest object of desire? What is the most outstanding virtue? Drummond's rejoinder to all these questions is the same. He believes that the greatest thing in the world is love.

Drummond says that "Love itself can never be defined because it has so many different parts." He compares love to light. He says that when a scientist passes an ordinary beam of sunlight through a crystal prism, it comes out on the other side, broken up into its component parts of red, blue, yellow, violet, orange, green, purple, and all of the other tints and hues of the rainbow. He believes that this same kind of analysis is obtained by passing the compound of love through the prism of inspired intellect. Henry Drummond concludes that real love is found in the following nine virtues listed below:

1. Love embodies patience
2. Love exemplifies kindness
3. Love includes generosity
4. Love demonstrates humility
5. Love reacts with courtesy
6. Love reflects unselfishness

7. Love maintains an even temper

8. Love is guileless, seeing the good in others

9. Love manifests sincerity

I believe that love personifies all the virtues listed above. Consequently, I strongly believe, along with Henry Drummond, that love can be a vital, powerful force in our lives, bringing meaning to and enriching our existence. Robert Browning echoed this belief when he said, "Love is the energy of life."

With that in mind, I suggest that we examine five relationships where the mastery of love's elements can make a tremendous difference in the quality of our lives.

Relationship with Self

I agree with this statement from an anonymous author: "Love yourself and your life and then you can love others." The solid basis for having a positive, loving relationship with others is to have a positive, loving relationship with yourself.

Psychologists tell us that there are basically two references of thought by which individuals value themselves. They see themselves as valuable and worthy of love according to "doing" or "being."

People who values themselves according to a "doing" frame of thought love themselves according to the things they do. For instance, human beings, using this reference, would see themselves of value and worthy of love if they earned a certain salary, or if they weighed a certain amount, or if they were married or in a long-term relationship, etc. The problem with using the "doing" framework for self-evaluation is that there are numerous variables, subject to change, beyond our control. If you only love yourself according to your paycheck, what happens if you lose your job? If you only value yourself according to your physical condition, does your appraisal of yourself change with each pound lost or gained? If you have to have a significant other or be part of a pair to see worth in yourself, how do you feel about yourself if that relationship ends?

In *Cool Runnings*, a movie about the first Jamaican bobsled team, the team's leader, who was driven to copy the Olympic medals achieved by his father, asked their gold medalist coach what it was like to receive a gold medal. The coach, who realized that the team leader saw Olympic medaling as a life-defining moment, responded with some very wise counsel for all "doing" self-evaluators. He said, "If you're not enough without it, you'll never be enough with it."

Those who love themselves according to a "being" viewpoint, see themselves as having an intrinsic worth. They recognize that they are children of God, that they have inherent talents and abilities, that they have the power of choice and decision, and that they, in and of themselves, are worthy of love.

This doesn't mean that they feel validated in being cocky or arrogant. This doesn't mean they view themselves as "A-Okay: No Change Needed Here." Instead, it means that, while they recognize areas where they need to improve and grow, they are gentle and kind with themselves, forgiving when they falter, seeing themselves as capable of ultimate success. They have a quiet, unshakable confidence in who they are.

Those who love themselves according to a "being" viewpoint have a better emotional framework for reaching out to and loving others. Jane Roberts encourages, "You must love yourself before you love another. By accepting yourself . . . your simple presence can make others happy."

I had a patient, whose weight had ballooned to 600 pounds. At that point in his life, he was totally bed-ridden, unable to move about or function normally. He loved himself enough, however, that he was determined to do something about it. He has now lost 360 pounds and is living a productive life. He told me that in order to survive the future, we have to go back to the past.

I truthfully believe that we can all benefit from this man's insightful advice. If we want to have a productive future, we do need to go back to the past. We need to determine how and when we developed a "doing" evaluation of ourselves. We need to change our thought patterns, visualize our intrinsic value, and learn to love ourselves. Lucille Ball summarized it best when she said, "Love yourself first and everything else falls into line."

Relationship with Spouse

An interesting sociological offshoot from the September 11th tragedy was a spiked increase in marriages. At first glance, this seems like an anomaly. However, upon careful reflection, it is easy to understand the reason behind this behavior. The September 11th terrorist attack on home soil was devastating for all Americans, throwing us emotionally off-balance. What better and more productive way to recover from an act of vicious hatred than to step forward into committed love.

Scientists have long realized that marriage has its benefits. Research has shown that a happy, committed marriage is a great anti-aging tool.

Todd E. Linaman, Ph.D. in his article "Marriage Does Have Its Benefits!" reports the following facts research has uncovered about the married state:

- Married people live up to eight years longer than divorced or never-married people (Murphy et al., 1997).
- Married people are much happier and likely to be less unhappy than any other group of people (Waite, 2000).

- The incidence of mental illness is lower in married people as compared with unmarried or divorced people (Waite, 2000).

- Married people suffer from long-term illnesses much less than those who are unmarried (Murphy et al., 1997).

- Married men are more financially successful. They earn 10-40 percent more than unmarried men (Waite and Gallagher, 2000).

- Married people save more. Couples in their 50's and 60's have a net worth per person almost double that of divorcees, widows, or other unmarried people (Smith, 1995).

- Married people are less likely to engage in unhealthy behaviors such as drug and alcohol abuse.

- People who are married have twice the amount of sex as single people and report greater levels of satisfaction in the area of sexual intimacy.

In his article, Linaman stresses that marriage isn't easy, and that the benefits of marriage are not achieved effortlessly. He states that "if you have been married for more than a week you know how challenging and difficult marriage can be." I agree with Leo Buscaglia's assertion that love, "like any other living, growing thing . . . requires effort to keep it healthy," and I know that the benefits of marriage are worth the effort it requires. The following three suggestions for having a vital, fulfilling, beneficial marriage may be helpful.

Commit Completely
"Dance like no one is watching; love like you'll never be hurt."—Anon.

Joan Borysenko, Ph.D. states that "the soul grows well when giving and receiving love." She counsels that you should nourish your soul daily "by loving others and being vulnerable to their love." Linaman points out that a strong commitment netting the benefits of marriage is easiest "to maintain early on when the relationship is characterized by closeness and romantic love." He warns, however, that following this phase, every normal marriage moves into a "period of disappointment and disillusionment brought on by the normal stressors of marriage, unmet expectations and the undeniable reality that one's partner has faults. In other words," he says, "the rose-colored glasses become clear." Partners in every successful marriage make a conscious choice to honor the marriage commitment they have made. I share Henri De Montherlant's belief that "we like someone *because*. We love someone *although*."

Love Lovingly

"To be loved, be lovable." —Ovid

A mistake that is commonly made is viewing love as simply a feeling, implying no effort needed. There are those who talk of falling in and out of love as if there is no choice in the matter. Love is a choice. I support Stephen Covey's statement: "Love—the feeling—is a fruit of love, the verb." We need to make the choice to be lovable and to treat our spouse with love.

Bernie Siegel shares the following advice for developing loving characteristics, paraphrasing something the anthropologist Ashley Montagu once said:

> The way I change my life is to act as if I'm the person I want to be. This is, to me, the simplest, wisest advice you can give anyone. When you wake up and act like a loving person, you realize not only that you are altered, but that the people around you are also transformed, because everybody is changed by the reception of this love.

Delight in Differences

"What counts in a good relationship with others is not so much how compatible you are, but how you deal with incompatibility." —*George Levinger*

As youth gaze down the road of life at marriage in the distance, they dream of meeting a soul mate and knowing complete compatibility. Maturity, on the other hand, looks at marriage realistically and seeks not so much for total compatibility, but rather for understanding and love. This concept is beautifully illustrated in the following story:

> As a teenager I had certain ideas in my mind that constituted the idyllic life of love and marriage. In Home Economics our teacher had us plan the perfect wedding and the perfect reception right down to the throwing of rice and driving away in a limousine. It was just like the movies where the nice guy gets the beautiful girl, and they live happily ever after. Reality was not a part of the picture.
>
> After high school came college and my determination to become a nurse. I forgot about marriage. I could put that on hold for now. I was going to help people and travel.
>
> Surprisingly, two years later I met the man I would marry. It's often said, "opposites attract." This was certainly true about us. He was from a small town in Idaho and farmed with his father. I was from a Southern town, which had a greater population than the entire state of Idaho. I had always been emphatic that I didn't know whom I would marry, but one thing I knew for sure was that he would NOT be a farmer or a dairyman. Well I was wrong on both counts. My husband and his father were farmers and dairymen.

We were married in October just prior to the beginning of heavy snowfalls. By December we were walking on crusty snowdrifts over the tops of fence posts. Chains for the snow tires were required most all winter. Our only entertainment was listening to the radio or attending the local high school sporting events.

My new husband was a lover of sports. He had been a champion boxer and also participated in most sports. I was a lover of the arts, speech, drama, and dance. The nearest town with this kind of entertainment was forty miles away, and the highway was closed off and on all winter long.

We had only been married seven months when I received word that my mother, who had been battling cancer, could not live much longer. Even though there was the dairy with 75 cows to care for and the farm with 1400 acres to be worked, when my husband read the telegram, he didn't hesitate. He immediately said, "Honey, get your bags packed while I make reservations for you. Your place is with your mother and your father right now." To my new husband, there had been no other decision to make.

Every week I would receive a letter from him telling me all about how the farm was doing and inquiring about my parents and me. Little was said about his sadness of being alone or of missing his new bride except at the very end of each letter, where an unmistakable "I love you" was written. Teenage dream letters would have been filled with remarks of undying love and the pain of missing me, but his letters were simple words of our reality together.

Four months later, after the funeral was over and final matters were taken care of with my father and brother, I returned to Idaho where I knew my husband would be at the airport to meet me. The look in his eyes told me more than any dream letter could have. The joy and honesty of love was deeply represented on his face.

On the 80-mile drive to our home, I talked incessantly while he quietly listened, without interrupting. When he finally had a chance to respond, he asked me to open the glove compartment of the car and take out an envelope with my name on it. "I wanted to give you something special to let you know how much I missed you," he said quietly. I opened the envelope to find season tickets for both of us to all the participating fine art functions within an 80-mile radius of our home. Our income was not substantial, and I was stunned. "I don't believe this," I argued. "You don't enjoy these things!" When I finally stopped protesting, he reached out, hugged me, and quietly said, "No, but you do, and I will learn."

In that moment, I realized marriage wasn't always a 50/50 proposition. Sometimes real love operated on a 100/0 ratio. I understood from my husband that love means putting your spouse first. His example taught me a great lesson, a lesson that has made for a happy marriage for over 51 years.

Benjamin Franklin assured, "Those who love deeply never grow old. They may die of old age, but they die young."

Relationship with Family

A boomerang is an interesting object. To those familiar with the technique of boomerang tossing, it is an easy matter to throw a boomerang high into the air and have it come right back to you. To the novice, getting a boomerang to return to you is far more difficult and requires far more effort than you'd ever dream possible.

Likewise, love is an interesting entity. To those conversant with the realities of love, it is not hard to offer humble, unselfish, sincere love, realizing that through patience and sustained love, it will be returned to you tenfold. To the uninitiated, however, selfishness and immaturity can make love seem far more challenging and demanding than you'd ever dream possible.

I firmly believe that in family relationships love is an essential ingredient. I know that if you give love, you receive love. After Mother died, I lived next door to my uncle and aunt. Theresa Neve, my mother's sister, became a surrogate mother to me. Other than my mother, she is the sweetest, most inspirational person I've ever known. Aunt Theresa, now almost 80 years old, has always referred to me as Little Jim to distinguish me from my father. Every other Friday when I have office hours in New Castle, a location near my aunt's home, I go visit her. She seems to enjoy my visits, and I know I do. Despite advanced age and health problems requiring dialysis, Aunt Theresa makes pizza, sauce, and a care package for her middle-aged "Little Jim" to take home. As much as I appreciate her cooking, I value her love and devotion even more. Aunt Theresa stepped in and filled the hole left in my life with the death of my mother.

Victor Hugo once said, "the supreme happiness of life is the conviction that we are loved; loved for ourselves, or rather, loved in spite of ourselves." In the best family circumstances, this need for unconditional love is met completely and fully.

We need to realize that this kind of family love and support takes time and effort. "Quality" rarely supercedes "quantity" when referring to the amount of time needed for family interaction. John Crudele illustrated this concept very clearly when he said "kids spell love T-I-M-E."

Enduring, loving, supportive family relationships do take work. But the time and effort spent in forging those family ties are well worth it. I often told my daughter Brooke that my mother was the inspiration of my life. I wanted my daughter to realize what a wonderful woman her grandmother was. On Father's Day this past year, Brooke gave me a card, and when I read it, it brought tears to my eyes. She had written, "Dad, I just wanted you to know something. I love you every bit as much as you love your Mother."

Relationship with Humanity

The benefits of love are not limited to those who are happily married or have strong family relationships. To reap the benefits of love described above, we just need to be involved with others in general. To paraphrase a familiar song lyric, research has discovered that "people who need people are the [longest-living] people in the world."

John Donne, an early 17th Century metaphysical poet, wrote a famous essay regarding our relationships with others. During a period of time when Donne was quite ill and painfully aware of his own mortality, he was lying in bed when he heard the village bells start to ring. He realized that the bells were used to signal a death had occurred. Donne, wondering who had passed away, thought of the sorrow the family must be feeling and questioned if this loss would impact his life. Later, in a reflective state of mind, remembering his thoughts at the time, Mr. Donne penned these words:

> No man is an island, entire of itself; every man is a piece of the continent, a part of the main. If a clod be washed away by the sea, Europe is the less, as well as if a promontory were, as well as if a manor of thy friend's or of thine own were: any man's death diminishes me,

because I am involved in mankind, and therefore never send to know for whom the bells tolls; it tolls for thee.

Karl Menninger stated, "Love is a medicine for the sickness of the world; a prescription often given, too rarely taken." I believe if we have the courage to take the medicine prescribed above, we will certainly reap the benefits.

Clearer Vision

Helen Keller said, "As selfishness and complaint pervert and cloud the mind, so love with its joy clears and sharpens the vision." I learned a lesson about this type of vision from a colleague whom I look up to and respect, Dr. Joel Swansen. I would characterize Dr. Swansen as one of the brightest, nicest, most sensitive, and caring people that I've ever known. One day Dr. Swansen said to me, "You know the world is full of magic. Sometimes you just have to close your eyes and look for it." I realized the truth of that statement. There is magic in the world—magic inside of every person we meet and with whom we interact. Sometimes we just have to close our eyes and use our heart and the power of love to capture the magic of life and to really "see" clearly. As Antoine De Saint-Exupery counseled, "It is only with the heart that one can see rightly; what is essential is invisible to the eye."

It is my belief that as we reach out to others, we will find ourselves better able to rise above the challenges and hardships of everyday living. I sincerely support Sophocles' statement, "One word frees us from the weight and pain of life; that word is love." But, loving others doesn't just help us cope with life's challenges, it also helps us find meaning and purpose in the attempt.

Find Meaning and Purpose in Life

By being lovingly involved in humanity, we are able to achieve man's noblest aim, which is to make a positive difference in the world. At the start of the Christmas classic, It's a Wonderful Life, the central character George is wallowing in feelings of failure and self-pity. He feels the world would be a better place if he had never existed at all. Through the help of an angel named Clarence, George comes to realize that his life has had purpose and meaning—that he has made a difference.

Emily Dickinson enumerates the ways, through love, that each of our lives can make a difference. She writes:

> If I can stop one heart from breaking,
> I shall not live in vain;
> If I can ease one life the aching,
> Or cool one pain,
> Or help one lonely person
> Into happiness again,
> I shall not live in vain.

I truly believe love is one of the defining elements of the "forever factor." As we incorporate love with all its parts into our lives, we will live longer, more contented lives.

Forever Facts:

You can't love others until you love yourself.
Marriage has its benefits.
Act like the person you want to become.
Although not always the easiest of relationships, family interactions are without doubt some of the most important.
Love gives meaning to life.

"If you haven't got any charity in your heart, you have the worst kind of heart trouble."
—*Bob Hope*

Finding Yourself

A wise man once said: "We have been given two hands—one to receive with and the other to give with. We are not cisterns made for hoarding; we are channels made for sharing." I believe that a life of value is based on a sincere interest in and concern for others. I can personally testify that as you implement that concern in helpful, supportive ways you not only help those you serve, but you bring joy to yourself, as well.

There was an article about unselfish service that appeared several years ago in popular magazine. The author emphasized that gracious giving requires neither special talent nor large amounts of money. He said that the only requirement for giving is for the heart and head to act together, expressing real feelings.

Emerson points the way for even the novice giver when he suggests, "The only gift is a portion of thyself." To plan a gift of "thyself" takes more thought than you might ordinarily use. With money, anyone can stop at a store and buy a gift. But when money isn't available, then time, effort, and creativity are essential. A young girl wanted to buy her mother a mother's day gift, but when she counted her money there just wasn't enough for what she considered a worthwhile gift for someone so special. Instead of buying something, she took some small boxes, which she tied with ribbon. Inside were slips of paper on which was printed, "Good for two evenings of baby sitting,

Good for two flower bed weedings, Good for three nights of dinner dish washing, etc." At her age, she had probably never read Emerson. Nevertheless, she had put a large part of herself into the small gifts.

When we serve others, we gain important blessings. Through service, we increase our ability to love. We become less selfish. As we think of the problems of others, our own problems seem less serious.

The well-known story of the Good Samaritan teaches us to help whomever is in need, whether they be friend or enemy. We learn from the compassion shown that there are important steps we should consider in giving service. First, we need to think past ourselves and notice the needs of others. We need to develop "window" vision, instead of "mirror" vision. Secondly, we shouldn't judge others. Usually, if we give people the benefit of the doubt, they'll surprise us. If we look carefully at those we might classify as our enemies, we might be surprised at the goodness, integrity, and compassion we find. Thirdly, we need to value all people, recognizing all have value and worth, regardless of race, creed, or financial standing. Finally, we should understand that service is not meant to take place only when it is convenient. Service should be given when needed.

When we consider the lives of people who serve unselfishly, we can see that they gain more than they give. One such person named Paul lost the use of both legs in an accident. Some men might have become bitter and useless, but Paul chose to think of others instead. He learned a trade and earned enough money to buy a house. There he and his wife made room for many unwanted and homeless children, some of whom were badly handicapped. Until his death twenty years later, Paul served these children and others in the community. In return, he was greatly loved. Paul turned away from his crippled legs, focusing on others. He forgot his own problems, and his life was enriched by the service he performed and the love that was returned to him.

We have probably all been taught the admonition "to lose yourself in the service of others." Too many of us, because of our own insecurities, have a tendency to turn inwardly, becoming selfish and complacent. Years ago in the Philippines, I recognized that we are here on earth to learn to turn ourselves outwardly, to lose ourselves through helping someone else, and to relieve personal disappointments by caring about the feelings of others.

John Rhodes once gave this wise counsel regarding our relationships with others:

"Do more than exist, live.

Do more than touch, feel.

Do more than look, observe.

Do more than read, absorb.

Do more than think, ponder."

The young woman in the following story is an example of Mr. Rhodes' advice in action. It was the holiday season. The young mother was experiencing financial difficulties. She struggled over how she would make her money stretch to take care of the presents for her young children as well as coming up with a Christmas gift for her parents. As she thought of her parents and the things they enjoyed, she came up with an idea. She went shopping and purchased inexpensive gifts that represented things her parents liked. She beautifully wrapped each gift, tied it with ribbon, and added a clever note to each present. As her parents opened the gifts, they were ecstatic. They unwrapped their favorite candy bar, nuts, a book by their favorite author, and more. It was so much fun to read each note, enjoying what their daughter had created just for them. The mother kept each of the notes for years and shared the idea with many friends.

Little did the daughter realize what her caring and cleverness would mean to her parents. When the other siblings would be visiting their parents on holidays and birthdays, and the daughter could not be in attendance, they always wanted her gift to be last one opened so they could, as one brother put it, "relish" her creativity from beginning to end. Truly, this young woman gave of herself to serve her parents.

We each need to realize that, throughout our lives, all of us depend on others for help. When we were infants, our parents fed, clothed, and cared for us. Without this care, we would have died. When we grew up, other people taught us skills and shared knowledge. Many of us have needed nursing care during illness, or money in a financial crisis. Since all have us have needed and received help at one time or another, each of us should be willing to repay help received by filling a need for others.

Some of us are content to ask God to bless suffering people, and then stand idly by doing nothing for them. In the Philippines, I witnessed untold poverty and suffering. When I saw the children with their physical deformities, I could have just prayed for them to get better. But, I knew I also needed to use the gifts God had given me and the medical skill I had acquired to help those children. I learned God helps others through us.

A widow tells of two children who came to her door shortly after she had moved to a new town. The children brought her a lunch basket and a note that read, "If you need anyone to do errands, just call us." The widow was gladdened by the small kindness and never forgot it. It is important that each of us examine the many ways we can help others regardless of our station in life. For example, we can donate money, food, or other articles to those who need them. We can be a friend to a newcomer. We can plant a garden for an elderly person or care for someone who is sick. We can take a flower by to brighten the day for a patient in a nursing home. All acts of service, both large and small, can be meaningful and make a difference in someone's life.

Service helps others. However, the greatest irony is that the person usually helped most in service is the person performing the service. I performed medical procedures for the Philippinos that they never could have paid for. This helped them; but, my service also blessed me. My life was enriched and my life's purpose was clearly defined because of this experience. When we lose ourselves in service to others, we more easily find ourselves because there is more of us to find. We are deeper, better people. George Granville summed up the value of service and its effect in our lives very succinctly, yet very effectively, when he wrote: "What we frankly give, forever is our own."

It is my hope that we each choose to experience the personal growth, peace, and joy that comes from reaching out to others. Because I know that, in the process, we will find ourselves.

Forever Facts:

Service keeps you young because it takes your mind off you and helps put your own problems into perspective.

A great way to serve is to volunteer somewhere. You could do anything from assisting an adult to read through a literacy program to entertaining sick children at a hospital to joining a political campaign to help a candidate you support get re-elected.

Local libraries are a good source for checking out volunteer opportunities, as well as social service organizations and churches.

Many organizations actively solicit for help. You could head up a March of Dimes collection campaign or you could ask for donations and walk to find a cure for cancer.

Look around your neighborhood. Sometimes you don't have to travel too far to find someone who could use your help. Maybe your neighbor could use your help in weeding his lawn. Maybe you could head up a neighborhood watch. Maybe you could plan a block party so all your neighbors could get to know each other.

Set some service goals. Determine to do one act of service a month or volunteer somewhere on a regular basis.

"Live! And be happy!"
—Carmelita Barber

Life Is Our Greatest Gift

My mother, Carmelita, taught me that life is our greatest gift, and, because it is a gift, we should make the most of it. I think most people want to be happy and to make a success of life.

Emerson defines success as:

> To laugh often and much, to win the respect of intelligent people and the affection of children, to earn the appreciation of honest critics and endure the betrayal of false friends, to appreciate beauty, to find the best in others, to leave the world a bit better—whether by a healthy child, a garden patch, or a redeemed social condition, to know even one life has breathed easier because you have lived. This is to have succeeded.

Ann Landers in her book, *Dear Abby, Dear Abby*, says:

> If you have a good name, if you are right more often than you are wrong, if your children respect you, if your grandchildren are glad to see you, if your friends can count on you and you can count on them in times of trouble, if you can face your God and say, "I have done my best," then you are a success.

One individual offered his definition for success and a

happy life as "freedom from fear, anger and guilt." Another said, "My life would be successful if I had good health and excessive energy."

Although success and happiness mean different things to different people, I maintain that to be happy and to attain any form of success, we must each reach out and embrace life. We must each make the most of this gift of life we've been given, and find the best in each and every day.

We sometimes live our lives from crisis to crisis thinking, "My life will be great as soon as I get this project done, or after the kids get married." We tell ourselves life will be better when we can trade cars or take a long vacation. Or we are sure life will be perfect when retirement comes. We can wish our lives away, hoping to find happiness in the next stage of life, expecting things to get easier down the road. The real truth is, there is no better time than right now to be happy.

Perhaps we should examine what brings happiness. Does it only come with possessions? Can you only be happy when others are doing things that please you? Or is happiness a choice—a way of looking at each and every day of this gift of life?

Maybe the question we should ask ourselves is, "If we're not happy now, then when?" There will always be a bump in the road of life or a detour we need to deal with. Life will always be filled with challenges.

Perhaps the following paragraphs will give us something to think about, and help to put the difficulties of life into perspective:

Some Facts About Grown-up Life

<u>First, the BAD news:</u>

Life isn't fair. The question isn't "Why me?" It's "Why *not* me?" No matter how nice and charming and bright and lovable you are, not everyone you meet is going to approve of you, or love you, or even like you. From time to time, it *will* rain on your parade. Every now and then, no matter how careful you try to be, you are bound to do something unbelievably stupid.

<u>Next the GOOD news:</u>

Unless you're hanging around with some really mean people, no one but you will remember the dumb things you've done. You do *not* have to have an opinion on everything. Virtually all of the bad "stuff" in life is survivable. A lot of it is even—eventually—useful. Although you're not nearly as wonderful as you hoped, you're also not nearly as terrible as you feared. I've never met a grown-up who, if given the choice, would choose to go back to being a kid.

— *Unknown*

Another perspective on life comes from Alfred D. Souza. He said, "For a long time it had seemed to me that life was about to begin—real life. But there was always some obstacle in the way, something to be gotten through first, some unfinished business, time still to be served, or a debt to be paid. Then life would begin. At last it dawned on me that these obstacles were my 'life.'"

Time waits for no one. So stop waiting till you lose 20 pounds, or gain ten pounds, or until your kids are on their own. Stop waiting for happiness to find you. Find happiness in every hour of every day. Look for the good. Regardless of how tough things seem today, keep in mind "this too shall pass."

Ralph Waldo Emerson put it this way, "If things are going good, enjoy it because it won't last forever. And if things are going bad, don't worry because it won't last forever either."

A reporter for a local newspaper asked a woman who was approaching her 100th birthday if she would like to share some thoughts about how to live a long, happy life.

The almost centenarian firmly replied:

> Yes, I would! Too many people are running around trying to find happiness, and they make remarks about living it up before they get old. My goodness, don't think about getting old. Just be happy whatever your age. Take care of yourself, stay healthy, and, when trouble comes (and it will), don't take time out to feel sorry for yourself or get angry. That takes too much energy. Study it out and ask the good Lord to help you. Be cheerful. Go in the kitchen and bake a big pan of cookies or something you can share with your neighbors. Then, if your neighbor wants or needs to talk, listen to her troubles, and you'll soon forget your own. That'll keep you young. You'll feel needed.

As an anti-aging physician, I realize that nobody grows old merely by living a certain number of years. People grow old by deserting their ideals. Years may wrinkle the skin, but to give up interest wrinkles the soul. Long, long years filled with worry, doubt, self-distrust, fear, and despair are what bow the head and turn the growing spirit back to dust.

General Douglas MacArthur shares these words of wisdom:

> Whatever your years, there is in every being's heart the love of wonder, the undaunted challenge of child-

like appetite for "what next," and the joy in the game of life. You are as young as your faith, as old as your doubt; as young as your self-confidence, as old as your fear; as young as your hope, as old as your despair. In the central place of your heart, there is a recording chamber. So long as it receives messages of beauty, hope, cheer and courage, you will be young. When the wires are all down, and your heart is covered with the snow of pessimism and the ice of cynicism then—and then only—are you old.

Many seek for a life of bliss deplete of problems, a life of continuous rapture, but religious leader Gordon B. Hinckley gives us the true version of a *good* life:

Anyone who imagines that bliss is normal is going to waste a lot of time running around shouting that he's been robbed. The fact is that most putts don't drop, most beef is tough, most children grow up to be just people, most successful marriages require a high degree of mutual toleration, and most jobs are often more dull than otherwise. Life is like an old-time rail journey— delays, sidetracks, smoke, dust, cinders, and jolts interspersed only occasionally by beautiful vistas and thrilling bursts of speed. The trick is to thank the Lord for letting you have the ride.

Remember that life is easier than you think. All you have to do is:
Accept the impossible,
Do without the indispensable,
Bear the intolerable, and
Be able to smile at anything.
—*Anonymous*

Life is *not* a spectator sport. In searching for the forever factor, I have found there are many anti-aging applications to try and healthy physical and mental changes to make. But the most important thing I've discovered is that to utilize the forever factor, we have to start *TODAY*. The day after tomorrow just isn't soon enough. To make the most of this gift of life, we have to start *NOW* to "**LIVE! AND BE HAPPY!**"

Forever Facts:

Every day you are getting older. There is no time to start work on anti-aging like the present.

Happiness is not an achievement, it is a state of mind.

"Never leave that till tomorrow which you can do today." — *Benjamin Franklin*

APPENDIX

Determining Your Biological Age

1. Do you have reduced lean body mass?

2. Do you have increased body fat?

3. Do you lack a positive sense of well being?

4. Do you have reduced energy and vitality?

5. Is your waist measurement greater than it was ten years ago?

6. Is your hip measurement greater than it was ten years ago?

7. Do you notice reduced muscle strength over the past ten years?

8. Do you notice a reduced ability to exercise?

9. Do you notice increased level of depression?

10. Do you feel increased levels of anxiety over the past decade?

11. Have you experienced a have reduced mental performance over the past decade?

12. Do you feel stressed-out at times?

13. Are you generally pessimistic about life?

14. Are you quick to get angry?

15. Do you have difficulty focusing and concentrating?

16. Do you look older than people your age?

17. Do you feel tired when you wake up in the morning?

18. Are you less social than in the past?

19. Have you noticed a decline in your sexual performance?

20. Do you have trouble sleeping?

21. Does it take longer for you to fall asleep?

22. Do you have more difficulty thinking clearly and remembering?

23. Do you have decreased HDL cholesterol?

24. Do you have an increased LDL cholesterol?

25. Do you have a deficiency in DHEA or melatonin?

26. Has your vision diminished over the past decade?

27. Has your hearing diminished over the past decade?

28. Does it take a long time for you to get over a cold or flu?

29. Does it take a long time for cuts or bruises to heal?

30. Is your blood pressure borderline or high?

31. Do you suffer from indigestion?

32. Do you often fail to have regular bowel movements?

33. Do you get up at night to urinate?

34. Are you slowly losing your hair?

35. Do you have food or inhalant allergies?

36. Do you have white spots on your fingernails?

37. Do you have longitudinal ridges on your fingernails?

38. Do your fingernails appear thin and weak?

39. Do you have more headaches than a decade ago?

40. Do you have cold hands or feet?

If you answered **"yes"** to more than **ten** of these questions, your biological age is the same or greater than you chronological age.

If you answered **"yes"** to more than **half** these questions, there is a large gap between your biological age and your chronological age—indicating your body is **aging too fast.**

Ideally, we want to set a goal to lower our biological age 10, 20, or even 30 years below our chronological age.

Above chart taken from the book *Quantum Longevity* by Paul Yanick.

The Future is Now

At the beginning of the 20th century, most people were not expected to live past age 48. Today, the average life expectancy in the United States is officially listed at 78, although it is not unusual to find people going strong into their 80's.

Dr. Ronald Klatz states in his book *Grow Young with HGH*:

Within the next thirty years, we can expect to see life spans of 120–130 years accompanied by good physical and mental health. The use of antioxidants, such as co-enzyme Q10, vitamin C, vitamin E, and the carotenoids, which actually get at a root cause of aging, the free radicals that ravage the cells and cellular components, will help prevent and delay heart disease, cancer and a host of other diseases and could add another ten years of functional life to the average life-span.

In the next five to ten years we can expect to see:

- Cardiac treatments, such as totally implantable artificial hearts, modified heart assist devices, and fetal cardiac cell transplantation, which will grow revitalized heart tissue.

- Biomarker assessments of the rate of human aging which will allow anti-aging specialists to monitor each patient's progress to slow the speed of biological aging and enable researchers to pick out the drug or therapy that is most effective in inhibiting or reversing the aging process. This advance should increase the average human life span in the United States to 85 years.

- Blood tests which will screen for biochemical markers of DNA damage and early cancer growth. This will lead to detection of most cancers at a time when they are more than 90 percent curable.

In ten years, based on the most advanced concepts of today, we can expect to see:

- The Human Genome Project, which has completed more than 90 percent of its goal of mapping all the human genes, rocketing genetic therapy to the forefront of clinical medicine.

- Effective treatment for Alzheimer's disease and age-associated loss of memory and cognition, which will include drugs to improve mental processing, speed, and memory retention.

- Nanotechnology, atom-by-atom construction, which will yield molecule-sized instruments and computers much smaller than a human cell, allowing nanosurgeons to correct almost any biological malady or anatomical defect.

- Advent of cloning techniques that will support body part replacements.

The scientific breakthroughs listed above are awe-inspiring feats of modern medicine that will, without doubt, extend and improve the quality of life for millions.

It is not necessary. however, to sit around waiting five to ten years for these technological advances in order to improve our lives. Until the above techniques are ready and available, we can take charge of our own lives and extend and improve our quality of life through self-education by studying, learning, and applying principles of anti-aging medicine.

In this book, Dr. Barber has given us information, inspiration, and encouragement to help us visualize the possibilities of anti-aging and to commit to living a younger, healthier lifestyle, gearing us up to successfully fight against the disease of aging.

In his upcoming book, *The Ageless Future: Ninety Days to the Forever Factor*, Dr. Barber will detail a 90-day program for achieving the "forever factor." He will share the latest expert advice in such fields as nutrition, exercise, skin care, healthy sex, aesthetic surgery, positive mental attitude and stress management that will allow us to take specific steps to arm ourselves against aging. Building on the foundation of his first book, Dr. Barber will map out an age specific 90 day agenda to enable his readers to take charge of their aging process. He will list day-to-day activities for all ages that will slow and reverse the signs of aging.

The future is now. Each day more scientific information is being discovered to help each one of us live longer and better lives. Dr. Barber is committed to sharing anti-aging breakthroughs that will help us find success in our search of the "forever factor."

*Many other resources about the fight against aging are available at **www.foreverfactor.com***

Bibliography

Armstrong, Herbert. *The Plain Truth (Mystery of the Ages)*. New York: Dodd, Mead, 1985.

Backman, Robert L. *Be Master of Yourself*. Salt Lake City, Utah: Deseret Book Company, 1986.

Barrera, Regina. *They Used to Call Me Snow White—But I Drifted: Women's Strategic Use of Humor*. New York: Viking, 1991.

Berger, Stuart. *Forever Young*. New York: Morrow, 1989.

Bolander, Donald O. *The New Webster's Quotation Dictionary*. Lexicon Publications, Inc., 1987.

Carper, Jean. *Food, Your Miracle Medicine*. New York: Harper Collins, 1993.

Carper, Jean. *Stop Aging Now*. Thorndike, ME: G.K. Hall, 1996.

Casper, Dorothy Jean Small. *Blueprint 4 Living Newsletter*. Weekly Online Newsletter. [Blueprint4Living@bizland.com]

Cousins, Norman. *Anatomy of an Illness*. New York: Bantam, 1981.

Cool Runnings. Dir. Jon Turteltaub. Walt Disney Video. Distributed by Buena Vista Home Video, 1994.

Crowley, Geoffrey. "Stress Busters: What Works." *Newsweek*, 14 June, 1999.

Dead Poets Society. Dir. Peter Weir. Touchstone Home Video, 1990.

Frankl, Vicktor Emil. *Man's Search for Ultimate Meaning.* New York: Insight Books, 1997.

Gandhi. Dir. Richard Attenborough. Columbia TriStar Home Video, 1982.

It's a Wonderful Life. Dir. Frank Capra. Monarch Home Video, 1989.

Journal of the American Medical Association. Editorial. January 1988 edition.

Klatz, Ronald. *Grow Young with HGH.* New York: Harper Collins Publishers, 1997.

Lamm, Steven. *Younger at Last.* New York: Pocket Books, 1998.

Lineman, Todd. "Marriage Does Have It's Benefits." Family Life Communications Incorporated, 2002.

Mackoff, Barbara. *What Mona Lisa Knew.* Los Angeles: Lowell House, 1990.

Mahoney, David J. & Restak, Richard. *The Longevity Strategy.* New York: Dana Press, 1998.

Maltz, Wendy & Larry. "Healthy Sex CERTS Model." Maltz Counseling Associates, 1996. [http://www.healthysex.com]

Manton, Kenneth G. *Statistical Application.* New York: J. Wiley, 1994.

Nied, Robert J. "Promoting and Prescribing Exercise for the Elderly." *American Family Physician.* Feb. 2002 issue.

Packer, Lester. *The Antioxidant Miracle.* New York: Wiley, 1999.

Pauling, Linus. *Vitamin C and the Common Cold.* San Francisco: W. H. Freeman, 1970.

Pottker, Janice. *Dear Abby, Dear Abby.* New York: Dodd, Mead, 1987.

Rocky. Dir. Robert Chartoff. MGM/UA Home Video.

Rosenfeld, Albert. *Prolongevity.* New York: Morrow, William, & Co., 1983.

Schulze, Dr. Richard. *Common Sense Health and Healing.* Santa Monica, CA: Natural Healing Publications, 2002.

Sears, Barry. *The Soy Zone.* New York: Regan Books, 2000.

Sill, Sterling W. *The Upward Reach.* Salt Lake City, Utah: Bookcraft, Inc., 1962.

Swenson, Richard A. *Margin.* Colorado Springs, Colorado: Navpress, 1992.

Thayne, Emma Lou. "Where Can I Turn for Peace?" *Hymns of The Church of Jesus Christ of Latter-Day Saints.* Salt Lake City, Utah: Deseret Book Company, 1985.

Whitaker, Julian M. *Shed Ten Years in Ten Weeks.* New York: Simon & Schuster, 1997.

Yanick, Paul. *Quantum Longevity.* San Diego, CA: ProMotion Publishing, 1997.

James J. Barber

Since 1986 Dr. James J. Barber has been Board Certified by the American Board of Plastic and Reconstructive Surgery. He graduated with honors in 1971 from the University of Pittsburgh, majoring with a premed curriculum. Dr. Barber was a member of Alpha Omega Alpha, the National Honor Medical Society, and the top graduate from Howard University's Medical School in 1980, graduating in three years.

He completed his surgical internship in residency at Cedars Sinai Medical Center in Beverly Hills, California in 1983. In 1985 Dr. Barber completed his plastic surgery training at the University of Texas in Houston, continuing with additional training at M.D. Anderson Hospital in Houston and at Rancho Los Amigos Hospital at the University of Southern California.

In addition Dr. Barber won the prestigious Spira award for excellence in creativity in plastic surgery. In 1985 he established his own plastic and reconstructive surgery practice in Pittsburgh, Pennsylvania. The doctor is still active as a surgeon and as an anti-aging physician.

Dr. Barber was one of the original physicians to join the Longevity Institute International in Montclair, New Jersey in 1995. In addition, he is a member of the American Academy of Anti-aging Medicine. Since 1995 he has been practicing anti-aging medicine and has established a substantial client base in this area.

In 1997 Dr. Barber founded a company with the purpose of developing nutritional supplements as a foundation for more advanced anti-aging therapy. The company's goal is to bridge the gap between basic health maintenance needs and more advanced anti-aging therapy.

Dr. Barber has made many public appearances in support of alternative modalities, including numerous cable and television features. He has also lectured throughout the country on anti-aging medicine.

Recently, Dr. Barber was honored by being named honorary co-chairman of the Physician's Advisory Board, and was given a national leadership award in that regard. Most recently, he was named as one of the nation's top plastic surgeons.

Dr. Barber is a devoted husband to his wife, Diane, of twenty-eight years and a loving father to his daughter, Brooke. He is also an avid sports fan and closely follows Pittsburgh area professional teams, as well as the University of Pittsburgh football and basketball programs.

A final note from James J. Barber, M.D.

With knowledge in anti-aging medicine doubling every 2.7 years, there is always new information coming to light on how to slow and even reverse the aging process.

To get the latest in anti-aging news and therapies, visit my website at **www. foreverfactor.com** and let me help you in your search for the "forever factor." I wish you well on your journey. Godspeed.